Social Skills and the Speech Impaired
Second Edition

Social Skills and the Speech Impaired

Second Edition

Lena Rustin and Armin Kuhr

with a contribution from Claire Topping

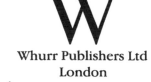

Whurr Publishers Ltd
London

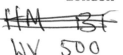

First Edition published by Taylor and Francis Ltd 1989
Second Edition published 1999 by Whurr Publishers Ltd
19b Compton Terrace
London N1 2UN
England

British Library Cataloguing in Publication Data available on
request.

ISBN 1 897635 56 7

Printed in the UK by
Athenaeum Press Ltd, Gateshead, Tyne & Wear

To Willie
for her constant help and support

Contents

Preface

Since publication of the first edition of this book, ten years ago, there has been an increasing awareness of the important role social skills play in communication. This encouraged speech and language therapists to embrace social skills training principles and intergrate them into their work in a wide variety of settings. The first edition of *Social Skills and the Speech Impaired* was well received by the profession and not only widely used both in the UK and USA but also translated into French, and a German edition is in preparation. The demand for an up-to-date resource has been high and so we were persuaded to revise the first edition. We hope that developments in theory and practice are well reflected in the new text.

Major revisions and extensions were undertaken in the chapter on *Cognition and Communication* since cognitive strategies are now extensively used in the treatment of a wide variety of disorders. *Principles and Elements of Training* has been expanded, particularly in relation to relaxation procedures. A chapter on *Group Therapy* has been added with an example of a *Group Programme* to help therapists to structure their group work by suggesting hierarchical therapeutic steps and linking them to specific exercises. As speech and language therapists now have an important role within educational settings, we invited Claire Topping to contribute a chapter on *Developing Social Communication Skills within the Mainstream School Context*.

We have also increased the number of exercises which we hope therapists will find beneficial.

Acknowledgements

We would like to express our grateful thanks to Willie Botterill for her invaluable contribution to the text; to Allison Nicholas for collating the exercises; to Rachael Rees, Isabel Brown, Rachel Farizman and Felicity Nichols for their speech and language specialist therapy advice; to Frances Cook for her help with the text and to Naomi Wood who so patiently typed the various drafts of the manuscript.

For ease of reading, therapists are referred to as being female and clients as male throughout the book.

Part I

Introduction

A substantial part of our lives is spent interacting with other people and the success or failure of these encounters can profoundly influence our development as individuals. In the social world in which we live we need the capacity to read social situations and respond appropriately to the myriad signals that human beings emit. This can mean the difference between popularity and loneliness and can smooth the route to professional and social success. We need others to satisfy both our emotional and biological needs and therefore person-to-person communication is one of the most essential human abilities. The demands of our society have become increasingly complex and there are many individuals who have found themselves without the skills necessary to cope with them. Social skills and assertiveness training evolved to meet the needs of those who lacked adequate models and learning opportunities to fulfil their social roles. Social skills, like other human skills, are gradually acquired in a number of ways. Children learn by imitating others and in particular parents provide important models on which a child bases his own behaviour. People are provided with models of appropriate and inappropriate behaviour in a variety of settings and these behaviours are observed and imitated. The acquisition of acceptable social behaviour can be impaired in cases of physical illness or emotional problems. A deficit in social skills might unduly exaggerate the consequences of disability, thereby starting a vicious cycle where physical or emotional problems reinforce each other and lead to the development of further social or psychological disturbances. Thus social skills training is based on the idea that skills are learned and consequently can be taught to those who lack them. The skills approach to the study of interpersonal behaviour has provided a useful conceptual framework that spawned productive research with fruitful clinical applications.

Original therapy programmes existed only for increasing assertiveness and reducing social anxiety. However, today, drawing on knowledge derived from studies in developmental, social and abnormal psychology, we not only know more about reasons for failure to acquire social skills, but also we have considerably improved our arsenal for treating social skills deficits in a wide variety of disorders.

The assessment and training procedures presented in this text reflect theoretical and practical developments in the field as well as benefit from our many years of clinical experience. The 'games' in the second part of the book, we hope, will be of direct practical use to therapists in treating a wide variety of communication disorders. The majority of published social skills programmes are geared towards linguistically able people and in many cases are not appropriate for speech and language impaired individuals. There is no 'cook book' approach to treating human problems, but behaviour therapy furnishes us with clear-cut suggestions of how to conceptualize problems and, depending on the specific goals, how to help clients to solve them.

The purpose of this book is to help speech and language therapists, occupational therapists, educators and other caring professionals in a practical way, increasing their efficiency by expanding their professional repertoire.

The book does not present a rigid approach but allows therapists both to improve their skills in assessing and identifying their clients' individual difficulties in social interaction, and to apply the necessary techniques, creatively adapted to the client, treatment setting and general resources.

Chapter 1
Fundamental Principles

Definition of Social Skills

The term 'social skills' seems to have been coined by the British social psychologist, Michael Argyle, when he explored analogies between human–machine and human–human interactions (L'Abate and Milan, 1985). Argyle recognized the limitations of applying a model based on perceptual and motor skills in relation to social behaviour but felt that despite its limitations, it was useful as a heuristic model.

Many processes are involved in the complex interaction of communication and there is no unitary measure or single theory of communication skill/social skill that would encompass all aspects of social communicative behaviour.

The term 'social skills' refers to the performance of behaviour in social interactions. A concise definition of 'social skills' tends to vary depending on the population it refers to, the environment in which the interaction occurred and the desired outcome of the interaction. For our purposes, social skills will delineate the repertoires of social behaviours including both implicit and explicit modes of communication that, when applied to social interactions, will tend to elicit social reinforcement and encourage positive interaction outcome. Furthermore, to be socially skilful implies the extent to which an individual can effectively draw on his repertoire of social behaviours to accommodate the endless variety of social situations in which interaction is essential.

The evolution of a precise definition of what constitutes social skills has been consistent with that of behaviour therapy in general. Social skills were seen as overt behaviours learned by observation and experience and the earliest definitions emphasized the observable nature.

Michelson *et al.* (1983) list six elements as defining features of social skills.

1. Primarily acquired through learning.
2. Comprise specific discrete verbal and non-verbal behaviours.

3. Entail effective, appropriate initiations and responses.
4. Maximize social reinforcement from others.
5. Interactive in nature, require appropriate timing and reciprocity of specific behaviours.
6. Influenced by environmental factors (age, sex, status).

A brief discussion of the term 'behaviour' is necessary when considering definitions of social skills. Behaviour in this context can refer to either the grouping of similar responses by breaking the behaviour down into its 'molecular' components (e.g. eye contact, head nodding, the words we use) or by grouping the behaviours according to their presumed function. These 'molar' categories would include assertion, co-operation and compliance. Sequencing, patterning and timing are other important aspects of behaviour.

We have to include the situations in which behaviours normally occur in order to understand the complete concept of social behaviour. The term 'situations' refers to the circumstances surrounding the behaviour of interest and is defined in terms of setting characteristics (e.g. home), degree of structure inherent in the setting (e.g. number of other people present) and the task or nature of the interactions.

Normally it will be quite difficult to operationalize the relevant parameters in a given situation, therefore it is necessary to be specific about the aspects that are important for each client group.

In order to look in detail at behaviours that would constitute social skills, lists were compiled to encompass all behaviours that contribute to social skills. These included skills such as observation, listening, speaking, meshing, expression of attitudes, social routines, tactics and strategies, non-verbal communication, reinforcement, questioning, reflecting, initiation and closure of contacts, explanations and self-disclosure. Some of these skills are more general than others and most of them can be broken down into their component parts; single elements such as looking, nodding, characteristics of speech. Hops (1983) criticized these compilations by observing that with the accumulation of social skills literature, a large variety of behaviours had been called 'social skills', rendering the term over-inclusive and no longer specifiable.

Despite these difficulties, many authors attempted to define social skills. Eisler, Miller and Hersen (1973), in the behaviouristic tradition, described socially skilled persons operationally as those who speak louder, respond more rapidly to others, give longer replies, evidence more affect, are less compliant, request more exchanges and are more open-minded in their expressiveness.

A more formal approach using the theoretical terminology of behaviour therapy was chosen by Libet and Lewinsohn (1973, p. 304) who defined social skills as '. . . the complex ability both to emit behaviours which are positively or negatively reinforced and not to emit behaviours that are punished or extinguished by others'. Neither of these definitions takes into account an important variable in interaction that Argyle (1982) called 'meta-perception'. This refers to the fact that interacting persons not only judge each other but are also concerned with how *they* are being judged and that this might significantly affect their behaviour. Perception of both the environment and one's own functioning in relation to the environment is important for understanding social skills.

In part we actively create our environment and, in turn, are influenced by it. We observe the actual situation we are in and our behaviours and modify them in the light of our reading of the external feedback and internal criteria, such as the desired outcome. This view of social behaviour emphasizes the importance of cognitive processes. Gambrill (1984, p.104) states that '. . . appropriate sequences of action related to particular situations are stored in our memory; socially competent people possess scripts for thousands of situations and employ them as relevant under the constraints of particular contexts — e.g. initiating a conversation at a party'. Therefore, we have to concern ourselves not only with the client's overt behaviour (e.g. rate and duration of eye contact) but also with the client's internal state (e.g. feelings, attitudes and perceptions). In keeping with the development of behaviour therapy, the cognitive aspects of social skills have also been incorporated into social skills training.

Cognitive processes refer to the generation of goal-directed aspects of skilled behaviour whereby the individual draws on his repertoire, reorganizing it according to the demands of the situation. This type of goal-directed behaviour requires:

- Decoding skills (receiving, perceiving, interpreting stimuli).
- Cognitive decision skills (generating appropriate response alternatives, comparing them with task demands, selecting the best response, searching the behavioural repertoire for this select behaviour, evaluating the utility of enacting the selective response).
- Encoding skills (execution of the selective response, including co-ordination of verbal, non-verbal, muscular and autonomic components; use of automatic or conscious self-monitoring of any discrepancies that might occur between intended and actual performance and using this information to initiate additional behaviour) (McFall, 1982).

Trower (1979, p.4) used cognitive concepts to describe socially skilled behaviour and focused on the qualitative outcome: '. . . the individual has goals or targets which he seeks in order to obtain rewards. Goal attainment is dependent on skilled behaviour which involves a continuous cycle of monitoring and modifying performance in light of feedback.

Failure in skill is defined as a breakdown or impairment at some point in the cycle . . . leading to negative outcome'. Trower's terminology — 'failure', 'negative outcome' — leads us to another important aspect of social skills training, i.e. the values that are implicit in training. Social skills training attempts to help the client to behave more 'skilfully'. In order to differentiate skilled and unskilled behaviour we have to establish criteria for socially desirable behaviours. Social norms change with lifestyles and educational background. An awareness of alternative social conventions and customs is necessary in order to keep an open mind about the goals an individual might choose.

There is a cultural difference in perspective between North American and European theory, research and practice in social skills training. In the United States, research on social skills basically grew out of the work of behaviour therapists (Wolpe and Lazarus, 1966) and social competence (Zigler and Phillips, 1961). However, in Europe the origins of research were quite different as they were based in social psychology and ergonomics (Welford, 1980). The Europeans view causes of social behaviour as being more internal. Furnham (1985) describes a general difference in the person–situation relationship, whereas the Americans are of the opinion that the organism is reactive to external social events — these being the primary causes of social behaviour. For a long time American researchers stressed assertiveness (practically being defined as synonymous with social skills) while the Europeans embraced a much wider concept. However, some basic principles are probably valid in most social classes and cultures. Grice (1967) maintained that in conversation contributions have to be informative, truthful, relevant and clear in order to be comprehensible. Although these rules are sometimes violated, they could still be used in relation to conversation skills and are particularly relevant for speech and language impaired clients. Despite differences in terminology, several parameters or dimensions of analysis appear across definitions and seem to be important in the conceptualizations of socially skilled behaviour:

- Interpersonal behaviour is emitted; it is goal directed, intentional to a certain degree, controlled by cognitions.
- These behaviours are identifiable and can be categorized.
- These behaviours can be learned (modelling, imitation, reinforcement).
- There are situational and social antecedents to the interpersonal behaviour.
- The behaviours are interrelated and synchronized.
- The characteristics of the participants in the interaction have to be taken into account.
- The behaviour is appropriate (implying a value judgement according to some criterion) to the situation in which it is employed.

We have identified several areas that need to be considered for an in-depth understanding of social skills. These are behaviours, cognitions, affects, and situational and linguistic parameters. We have also seen that the problem of definition is extremely complicated and that social behaviour is often ambiguous and defies operationalization. On a theoretical level the enormous complexities of an interactive model have not yet been mastered. There does not exist a scientific definition of social skills that is reliable and valid but this should not prevent us from developing sensible, coherent and effective training programmes. Furnham (1983) pointed out that in psychology there was an impressive accumulation of knowledge, *without* clearly defined concepts. We feel that the preoccupation with definition would be counterproductive if it stopped us from using and developing social skills training in our clinical practice.

Historical Background to the Origin and Development of Social Skills Training

Social skills training has been repeatedly criticized for its lack of a coherent structural and theoretical basis and this may be attributed to the many and varied sources from which it has developed. Social, applied, and cognitive psychology as well as behaviour therapy have served to augment the theoretical and practical application of social skills training.

Social Psychology

During the 1930s, the study of child development led to important theoretical, methodological and empirical contributions (Piaget, 1932; Moreno, 1953). One of the main areas of interest was children's peer relationships and their pro-social behaviours. Lewin and his colleagues focused on group dynamics and human interaction in groups (Lewin, Lippitt and White, 1939). This research later became one of the major building blocks of social skills (SS) training. More recently SS training has been broadened by the experimental work of social psychologists studying non-verbal aspects of communication and the structure of social situations (Hollin and Trower, 1986).

Applied Psychology

The major focus of industrial psychology was the analysis and evaluation of motor skill performance. It was only in the 1960s that social relations in industry were studied more closely, referring back to the earlier work of Lewin and his associates. The aim of this work was to improve communication between workers in order to gain higher levels of productivity. Welford (1980) cites Crossman (1960) as the researcher

who provoked interest in this facet of industrial psychology. Sub-
sequently, Argyle and Kendon (1967) published a paper drawing the
analogy between motor skill and social skill. The authors readily
acknowledged that this was definitely a simplification, yet it was a useful
paradigm in the early stages of social skills research.

Behaviour Therapy

Eysenck (1952) analysed outcome studies of psychoanalysis and came to
the conclusion that it was ineffective. His highly provocative article instig-
ated an in-depth discussion of the value of psychotherapy in general
which still continues (Grawe 1997). During this period behaviour
therapy began to develop, challenging the supremacy of psychoanalysis
by claiming that it was able to *prove* its effectiveness.

Behaviour therapy, which has important foundations in both learning
theory principles and experimental psychology, contributed substan-
tially to social skills training. Many techniques and the basic methodology are of behavioural origin. 'Assertion training' (Salter, 1949) bears
striking similarity to some of the social skills programmes in use today.
Shaping (reinforcing approximation of the final behaviour that is to be
developed) and token economy (manipulation of environmental contin-
gencies) are useful in social skills training as they facilitate the development of complex sequences of social behaviour. Social skills training
also benefited from later developments in behaviour therapy. Social
learning theory (Bandura, 1973; 1977) introduced cognitive processes
which were of substantial use to social skills training: modelling, imitation, self-reinforcement. Current social skills training packages, which
are aimed at the reduction of social anxiety, incorporate techniques used
in cognitive therapies (Juster *et al.*, 1997; Lucock and Salkovskis, 1988).

In the wake of behaviour therapy, social skills training was used in the
treatment of psychiatric disorders. Early work by Zigler and Phillips
(1960; 1961) highlighted the role of social functioning in recovering
from disorders such as schizophrenia. Recent research has confirmed
that a higher level of social competence correlates positively with shorter
hospitalization and a lower relapse rate (Falloon *et al.*, 1990; Hogarty *et
al.*, 1986).

Roff *et al.* (1972) and Cowen *et al.* (1973), having examined childhood
relationships and the preventive role of social skills training, were able to
show that the quality of children's peer relationships was predictive of
academic failure, antisocial behaviour and general psychopathology in
adolescence and adulthood.

Examination of the current state of social skills training reveals that it
has expanded rapidly over the last decade and a variety of programmes
for different populations have been developed. We may expect that the
many sources from which social skills training has evolved will continue

to influence and expand this field, thus perpetuating its creative and innovative, if unsystematic, development.

Rationale of Social Skills Training

From the moment of birth, parents are reacting to their infant as though he or she already had social motives. Very quickly parents develop definite perceptions of their child that are partially based on individual characteristics, the child's behavioural style or primary reaction pattern (sociability, distractibility, intensity of mood, activity, etc.). Infants who are 'difficult' will experience different maternal interaction patterns and less time in interaction with their mothers than will 'easy' babies (Brooks-Gunn and Lewis, 1985). We could therefore assume that children with physical and/or moral deficits will be treated differently by their parents. A lack of social stimulation, for instance, might lead to a deterioration in social behaviour, worsening the effects of the handicap (Matthews and Brooks-Gunn, 1984). Life and social interaction in the family during the early years lay the foundations for future developments and therefore are of great importance. The establishment of social relationships within the family and later outside the family is central to healthy, adaptive functioning.

Communication, usually accomplished through speech and language, is of the utmost importance in establishing and maintaining relationships. Language enables us to combine symbols into sequential units to express thoughts, intentions and experiences. It is an important vehicle by which we think, generate and express ideas. If children are unable to communicate verbally in the normal way, their chances of participating in satisfying interactions and forming good relationships are reduced. Doyle (1982, p.214) states that the '. . . ability to communicate verbally may be a very salient factor within the play choices of young children'. Young children normally seek out those peers with whom they are able to communicate verbally. Thus, the handicapped child could become isolated, restricting his opportunities to develop social skills. This might lead to behavioural problems which in turn would cause further isolation. Rubin and Ross (1982) report that it has been shown repeatedly that the perception of similarity is important from toddlerhood until early adolescence. Anybody who is different from his peer group will be less attractive and therefore his chances of normal social development would be diminished. A feeling of helplessness or hopelessness might develop from repeated social failures and result in avoidance of social situations and substantial social anxiety as well as depression.

If we look at human problems from this point of view, social skills training might be a way of breaking this vicious cycle. In order to change the quantity and quality of social interactions in children and adults with speech and language impairment, we have to conceptualize interpersonal failures as being founded in the 'learning history' of each individual. This will be dependent on the social and physical circumstances, the social norms and psychological expectations of the peer group and basic personality variables.

Social skills training for speech disordered individuals should aim at shaping language in form and content towards normality and by incorporating the pragmatic and functional aspects of communication to help them become as effective and as natural a communicator as possible within the constraints of their handicap.

A Process Model of Social/Communication Skills

Hargie *et al.* (1994) list six separate components of skilled social behaviour.

1. Goal directed: Communication is usually purposive or goal directed and success will be dependent on particular skills which require minimal effort and offer maximum efficiency.
2. Interrelated: Verbal and non-verbal elements of communication need to be closely synchronized.
3. Behaviour: Skills are made up of identifiable units of behaviour which an individual displays within a framework of knowledge, attitudes and abilities.
4. Appropriate: Competent communication requires the ability to meet the demands of specific individuals in differing social contexts. Behaviours must be within the boundaries and conventions of society and successful interaction will require both flexibility and adaptability.
5. Learned: Most forms of behaviour used in social interaction are learned and therefore can be improved where necessary. Learning when and how to communicate successfully is as crucial as learning the various techniques required.
6. Control: Skilful communication requires control over one's behaviour and competent timing of various elements of performance.

A process model of social skills includes cognitive, physiological and behavioural components. The main elements are as follows.

Situation

Social behaviour, in order to be effective, would need to be adapted to specific situations. It is important that each situation should be considered in terms of attainable goals, appropriate social rules, and knowledge that may be required. The relevance of this element is highlighted by a study by Mullinix and Galassi (1981) who looked at the content of

verbal interaction in assertiveness. They isolated four verbal components representing requests, each one more assertive than the last: (1) a
simple statement about conflict by two people; (2) adding a behaviour
change request; (3) adding empathy, and (4) adding a threat. Non-verbal
and paralinguistic behaviour were held constant. To the surprise of the
authors there was barely any difference between the effects of the
different behaviours. Obviously the simple dismantling of verbal
messages into basic ingredients is not enough and does not take care of
tacit general social knowledge and of situational components.

Goals/Plans

People can be ineffective communicators because they have inappropriate goals, are unable to identify clear goals or fail to plan how to
achieve them. It is important that one is responsive to feedback about
the effects of one's behaviour. Failure to respond appropriately to feedback can be caused by several factors including poor perception and
interpretation as well as emotional problems (see Figure 1.1).

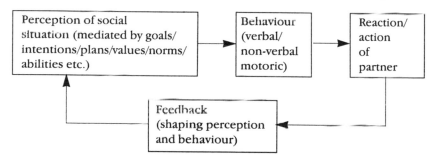

Figure 1.1: A simplified model of interpersonal communication

Perception: Effective communication requires correct observation and
interpretation of others' verbal and non-verbal behaviour. The ability to
perceive the points of view of others will enhance one's social interaction skills enabling us to respond and feed back successfully.

Self-presentation: How we present ourselves informs others about our
role, status and social position which will influence their reaction. Self-
presentation can 'go wrong' if it is misinterpreted by others.

Interpretation: We not only need to perceive the behaviour of others
correctly but must interpret it as well. Communication is a process
where we are constantly making decisions, sifting through information,
and deciding what is useful and needs to be acted upon. Accuracy of
perception and interpretation is partly dependent on knowledge of
language, values and rules relating to specific situations.

Reinforcement: One of the most important interaction skills is the ability to give and receive reinforcement. Offering high levels of positive reward encourages people to like us and to become more confident in themselves.

Both verbal acknowledgement, praise and non-verbal behaviours are required in reinforcing feedback. These non-verbal behaviours would include:

- Closer space.
- Touching.
- Head and body movements (nodding).
- Relaxed open body posture.
- Eye-contact.
- Positive facial expression (smiling).
- Moderate amount of gesture and animation as well as supportive para-language.

Flexibility, Creativity and Coping Skills

Successful communicators need to be highly flexible in order to accommodate all kinds of different situations and to be able to adapt their style accordingly. Creativity enables us to solve problems successfully, enlarging our choice of options. The ability to cope in a wide number of situations is essential and will be influenced by personal characteristics.

Ellis and Whittington (1981) identify four dimensions that are relevant for developing a training programme:

1. Inference: A low inference skill is easily observable and recordable whereas a high inference skill (e.g. sincerity) requires inferences to be made from behaviour.
2. Molecularity: Molecular skills such as mutual eye gaze are irreducible elements of interaction, whereas molar skills such as empathy or giving explanations are an amalgam of more molecular skills.
3. Specificity: Situation-specific skills are relevant and appropriate only in a limited range of situations, whereas generic skills are relevant in a great many situations.
4. Interactiveness: Some interactive skills explicitly require the person to mesh his or her behaviour with that of others.

On a more practical level Liberman *et al.* (1977) used a three-dimensional system as a guide to the practical content of social skills training:

1. Non-verbal behaviours: Eye-contact, facial expression, posture, gestures, loudness and tone of voice, pacing of speech, latency, duration of responding, fluency of speech.

2. Content of speech or conversation: Requesting something of another person, praising, thanking, complimenting, saying 'no' to an unreasonable request, going through a job interview, reacting appropriately to criticism, managing other daily instrumental and affectional encounters.
3. Reciprocity in communicating: Giving reinforcement to another to maintain conversation, initiating and terminating conversation, timing one's entry and exit from social groups.

Cognitive behavioural therapy has provided a host of valuable techniques that can be applied to social skills training, e.g. role play/rehearsal, modelling, feedback, instruction, homework assignments, relaxation, contingency contracts and cognitive restructuring. This repertoire enables therapists to develop training programmes that are applicable to a wide variety of speech and language impaired patients.

The emphasis on the positive educational aspects of treatment rather than the elimination of maladaptive behaviours calls for the detailed analysis of specific skill deficits in the individual repertoire (whatever the origin of this deficit, e.g. lack of experience, faulty learning, biological dysfunction).

Each client has different problems and needs. These have to be assessed in depth and then the individual programme (even if group treatment is provided) has to be designed. It is not yet possible to specify exactly how to match treatment procedures with clients to maximum effect but clinical experience and the accumulated knowledge on the effects of social skills training provide a good starting point. Scheidt and Schaie (1978) give an example of how to approach this problem empirically.

They sampled situations relevant for an elderly population. To describe these situations, four dimensions were selected and empirically tested: social/non-social, high/low activity, common/uncommon, supportive/depriving. The authors deduced from their studies that although the relevant behaviour strategies for these types of situations were different, they could be taught with the technique of cognitive restructuring.

Chang (1978) developed a 'situational control' of daily activity scale 'designed to measure the perceived personal control for a number of activities such as personal hygiene, eating and socializing'. This allowed the social skills trainer not only to identify problem situations but also to help elderly people recognize problems with their physical, mental and social state. The programme could then be tailored according to the needs of the structure and requirement of certain relevant situations. The work of Chang (1978) emphasizes not only the role of social perception — the ability to understand and process relevant interpersonal stimuli — but also that of intrapersonal self-monitoring.

Assessment techniques have become quite refined so that we are now better able to identify the focal factors that maintain the undesirable behaviour. If our intervention fails, our hypothesis is disconfirmed. We have, therefore, to look again at the problem, reanalyse it and alter our therapeutic strategy accordingly. This cycle is then repeated as often as needed to achieve the established goal.

The following major characteristics of behaviour therapy prevent a mere trial and error approach:

• Strong commitment to empirical evaluation of treatment and intervention techniques.
• Specification of treatment goals and procedures in operational terms and their measurement through different modalities (overt behaviour, cognitions, physiological reactions).
• Use of a problem solving approach geared towards generalization which is clear for clients and enables them to 'help themselves'.

To develop the instructional content of social skills training we might be aided by 'task analysis'. This is a procedure that is closely associated with behaviour modification technology. The objectives that are desirable for the client are specified in observable behavioural units. They are logically analyzed into component behaviours and broken down into a sequence of skill elements that comprise the behavioural chain which can then be arranged into a hierarchical framework. If the task analysis is performed well, it is possible to assess strengths and weaknesses of individual patients and design the content of their treatment programmes accordingly.

It is well documented that heightened emotional arousal might lead to a reduction in performance (Yerkes and Dodson, 1908). Most people know from their own experience that extreme emotions of fear and anger are likely to disrupt social behaviour. Even under normal circumstances, situations that are perceived as threatening, stressful or unpleasant (e.g. being the focus of attention, being rejected, a failure), might be anxiety-provoking and consequently negatively influence social performance. Not only is the global level of social skills important but also the type and structure of specific stressful social situations that clients normally encounter need to be incorporated into the assessment and training programme. This will enhance the ecological validity of the training situation, aiding generalization into everyday life.

The effectiveness of social skills training has been doubted in the past (Shepherd and Spence, 1983). This criticism seems to be still valid today as there are persistent methodological problems involved in coming to firm conclusions about the type of social skills training that is most effective for an individual client. On the other hand, there is considerable support now for the efficacy of social skills training in different patient groups.

Bellack (1987) used social skills training for chronic schizophrenic patients. He found that 'the effects of SST [social skills training] were not limited to changes on specific, narrow behaviour response components (e.g. eye-contact, voice volume)'. Additionally, 'the effects were discernible over and above the core everyday treatment program' and 'the effects were durable'.

Rustin (1984) tested the effects of social skills training on adolescent stutterers. She reported that 'the social skills only' group continued to feel more at ease at 12-months follow up than the 'technique only group', even though they were less fluent. They felt more confident in dealing with social interaction in spite of their stuttering.

In the past, the teaching of assertive behaviour would seem an obvious goal in therapy, as many anxious clients reported their feelings of helplessness and the sense of being pushed around by others. The benefits of assertion training have been widely recorded (e.g. Rimm and Masters, 1979), however, follow up of these clients showed that the effects of assertion training were not all pleasant or satisfying. Clients were perceived by their peers as lower in likeability, warmth, flexibility and friendliness (Kelly et al., 1980). Because of this, the concept of assertive training has been widened to social skills training and now to communication skills training, including the interdependence of social behaviour.

In order to expand our knowledge of social skills training, it would be helpful if therapists using this approach could collect data on their clients' progress, as this type of research will help to confirm social skills training as a reliable and valid method for preventing future psychological and behavioural distress.

It is clear that social skills training has its limitations and should not be expected to provide all the answers. Intensive, but relatively short periods of training should be seen as an addendum to other approaches rather than as a therapy in its own right. We feel that social skills training is a very useful therapeutic technique, specifically because of its adaptability and effectiveness. This potential will be realized if the training techniques are adapted to the specific client problems. Our endeavour is to guide therapists in the structure and function of social skills training in order to enhance the overall improvement of their client's communication.

Chapter 2
Non-Verbal
Communication
Behaviours

The focus of speech and language therapy intervention is often directed towards the deficits in verbal skills at the expense of non-verbal skills. The importance of non-verbal skills should not be underestimated. Birdwhistell (1970), one of the earliest authorities in the field of non-verbal processes in communication, estimated that in a typical dyadic encounter *verbal* components carry about one-third of the social meaning of the situation, while the *non-verbal* channel conveys approximately two-thirds. Non-verbal signals are more important that verbal behaviour in expressing feelings and attitudes (Argyle *et al.*, 1981) and they indicate how a message should be interpreted. If so much of the information we are transmitting and receiving is being conveyed via the non-verbal channel then it becomes essential to incorporate training of these skills within a speech and language therapy programme. Improvements in the non-verbal interaction skills of the speech and language impaired, despite the deficits in their verbal skills, should increase the effectiveness of their communication and in turn maximize the social reinforcement they receive from others. The consequent rise in self-esteem and confidence levels should also encourage an increase in their ability to initiate and maintain a conversational topic — skills which are vital to successful communication.

According to Dickson *et al.* (1993, p. 72) there are six main functions of non-verbal communication:

1. To replace speech. This happens in various situations, the prime example being sign language amongst the profoundly deaf. However, in many contexts a meaningful glance, a caring touch or a deliberate silence can be an adequate substitute for a verbal message.
2. To complement the verbal message. In most instances this is the main function of non-verbal behaviour. If we say we are happy, we are expected to look happy.
3. To regulate and control the flow of communication. Turn-taking during conversation is controlled by non-verbal signals. This is indic-

ated by stopping speaking, raising or lowering the final syllable and looking directly at the listener.

4. To provide feedback. It is necessary to monitor the non-verbal reactions of others during social encounters in terms of whether they are still listening, are worried, and/or have understood what has been said. We need to be sensitive to others' non-verbal feedback and be able to interpret this information whilst also being aware of our own non-verbal feedback.

5. To help define relationships between people. This facilitates identification and prevents role confusion between people.

6. To convey emotional states. It is generally agreed that emotions are primarily recognized through non-verbal behaviour. This is an important function since saying to someone 'I dislike you' may lead to overt aggression, whereas this message can be conveyed through subtle non-verbal cues, e.g. less eye-contact, turning the body away.

The importance of non-verbal interaction justifies its explicit inclusion in any social skills training and is particularly relevant to speech and language handicapped clients who often have specific difficulties coping with non-verbal cues.

The term 'non-verbal' includes all forms of human communication that are not controlled by the spoken word. However, an overlap exists in the paralinguistic aspects of speech, i.e. voice, rate of utterance and volume. These speech variations transmit extremely important information to the listener and therefore have to be considered in depth. Other non-verbal information is transmitted by body movement (stiff posture might suggest tension or anxiety); facial expression (may display emotions); and physical appearance (age, sex and including any possible visible handicaps).

Non-verbal behaviour serves important functions for both cognitions and affects. Whether a child's answer to a question is 'yes' or 'no', can be conveyed as effectively by a nod of the head or a smile as by a verbal response. It can be argued that non-verbal behaviours are frequently even more effective than verbal responses in influencing a person's judgement about the true meaning of an utterance. It is widely believed that non-verbal responses are less easy to control voluntarily than are verbal responses; as a result, a listener would be more inclined to accept non-verbal cues as being the true indicators of a person's position (belief, feeling, opinion.)

Anyone who visits a foreign country unable to speak the language will have experienced the power and the limitations of non-verbal communication. Perceptive individuals are able to identify, interpret and respond appropriately to a wide range of non-verbal cues with a fair degree of accuracy which helps them to adapt their behaviour and cope in difficult circumstances. However, this is not the case in less perceptive individuals, e.g. the speech and language impaired. Their difficulties with non-verbal cues compounds their problem, leaving them less able to cope as their speech disorder often dominates their attempts to communicate successfully. Thus, every social skills training programme and especially one directed at the speech and language impaired population should incorporate a component for the understanding and appropriate use of non-verbal behaviour.

There are generally accepted codes of conduct that exist within all social settings from the simplest to the most elaborate and these will vary from one cultural group to another. An understanding of these rules is essential as those who deviate from the commonly accepted patterns of behaviour disturb the social order and may precipitate some kind of social punishment.

Hargie *et al.* (1981, p. 24) use three categories to differentiate non-verbal behaviour:

- *Category 1:* Relatively rapidly-changing aspects of behaviour which include bodily contact, facial expressions, eye-contact, head nods and hand gestures.
- *Category 2:* Relatively stable aspects of behaviour which include posture, proximity, orientation, spatial behaviour, physical appearance and environmental factors.
- *Category 3:* Non-verbal aspects of speech which are referred to as paralanguage.

Rapidly Changing Aspects of Behaviour

Bodily Contact — Touch

Contact by touch serves mainly to establish and maintain social relationships. The type, intensity and frequency of bodily contact varies according to the situation, but touch tends to increase as a relationship develops producing a feeling of intimacy between individuals. It is important that touch given should complement the accompanying verbal message and that the gender of the recipient should also be considered. The range of emotions that may be expressed through touch is wide and may extend from feelings of warmth, caring, love and affection through fear and anxiety to aggression, punching and hitting. The intensity may also vary from the most intimate sexual relationship through very discreet and fleeting touches such as a friendly or comforting pat on the arm to a gentle touch on the elbow to direct or instruct others.

Facial Expression

This is one of the most important non-verbal means of communication. It can express emotional states from extreme happiness to great sadness and these feelings can often be reflected even when the person wishes to disguise them. Although the face can respond instantaneously and is an effective way of providing feedback, it can also be more easily controlled with regard to showing an emotional state. For example, a blank expression may hide a state of anger which can be shown by clenching fists and stiffening of body posture. If facial expressions and content of speech are not congruent, interpretation of emotional cues is more difficult.

Eye-Contact

Mutual gaze or eye-contact is used to regulate initiation and termination of communication as well as turn-taking. Eye gaze is an indication of a listener's attention and gaze aversion can be interpreted as an unwillingness to interact. Direct gaze may indicate dominance or aggression whereas gaze avoidance can be interpreted as submissiveness or shyness. There are cultural differences in the use of eye gaze which may cause misunderstandings between ethnic groups. In Western society the listener usually looks at the speaker about twice as much as the speaker looks at the listener (Argyle, 1975).

Gesture

Argyle (1969) found hand gestures to be second in importance to facial cues. They are sometimes the prime means of communication, as for the deaf population. Gestures may be used with or without verbal messages such as waving and pointing and can also denote emotional states, such as nail biting and foot tapping. Graham and Heywood (1976) found that when subjects were not permitted to use gesture when attempting to describe line drawings of two-dimensional shapes, their speech patterns were affected in terms of an increase in speech hesitancies and pauses. There are a range of meanings which may be associated with head movements. Slow head nods are usually taken that someone is listening and encouraging the speaker whilst fast head nods can be interpreted as showing impatience.

Relatively Stable Aspects of Behaviour

Posture

Posture can reflect a person's attitudes and feelings about himself and his relationship to others. It can also signify a person's emotional state. Anger can be emphasized by a tense posture whereas a feeling of warmth can be shown by a more relaxed stance towards a person. Impressions can be gained from a person's body position, i.e. the way he or she sits, stands or walks, and may convey a message of confidence or timidity.

Proximity or Personal Distance

While communication can convey information about relationships, some people require a greater space between them than others. Hall (1959; 1966) proposed four categories of interpersonal distance that are appropriate for north American and some northern European cultures:

1. Intimate distances: Expressing close intimacy such as making love, comforting or protecting. Distance between communicators from 6 to 18 inches.
2. Personal distances: Close personal relationships are reflected by a distance of 1½ to 4 feet.
3. Social or consultative distances: Business and professional – client interactions are denoted by a distance of 4 to 7 feet.
4. Public distances: These range from 12 to 20 feet. This would include public speaking where no recognition of being 'spoken to' is required.

To some extent, physical characteristics determine the amount of distance between people who are interacting. Kleck (1969) found that people communicating with physically disabled individuals chose a greater initial distance. Conversely, hearing impaired people are often more comfortable with closer proximity, particularly when using sign language. It seems that people of equal status tend to take up a closer distance with each other than people of unequal status. Individuals need to establish their own personal space as it enables them to maintain their dignity, respect and independence, which can become disturbed if this space is invaded.

Physical Appearance

Personal appearance serves to differentiate between people and conveys information regarding attitudes, status, personality type, occupation, etc. Judgements are made on the basis of a person's physical presentation and we manipulate appearance to fall in line with what we think is attractive. In a classic study, Lefkowitz *et al.* (1955) were able to illustrate the association between dress and perceived status and consequent differences in response behaviour. Pedestrians wishing to cross a road at a red traffic light were more likely to be influenced by a well-dressed person (high status) than by a poorly dressed one. Even small items of personal appearance may influence others. Thornton (1944) found that wearing glasses might produce a favourable judgement in terms of intelligence and industriousness. Facial appearance can also provide information regarding age and thus the appropriate level of interaction.

Environment

Social interaction is determined according to the physical environment; for example, one does not necessarily behave in the same way at home as in the office. There are different codes of behaviour that are appropriate in diverse settings and interaction will vary accordingly.

Paralinguistics

Paralinguistics is concerned with non-speech aspects of verbal communication, i.e. stress, tone, pitch, volume, rate, fluency and use of pausing. Paralinguistic signals can alter the meaning of what is said as well as how the message is received. The meaning of words may be contradicted by the tone of voice used. Paralinguistic cues are also used in forming judgements of others. Negative listener attitudes are often associated with low-volume, high-pitched voices of males and with husky, harsh, low-pitched voices of females (Hopper and Williams, 1973). Vocal cues also provide an indication of the emotional state of a speaker. Early studies by Fairbanks and Provonost (1939) demonstrated that fear, grief or anger were expressed with different vocal rates, pauses and pitch. Speaking loudly and rapidly with moderate-to-high pitch would convey the feeling of impatience. As well as signalling affect, the changes in a speaker's vocal pattern can be useful in gaining and retaining the attention of others. Sensitivity and flexibility will be required in terms of appropriate use of paralanguage.

Chapter 3
Cognition and
Communication

Introduction

During the 1970s behaviour therapy gained great popularity with numerous new techniques being developed and experimentally tested. By the end of the decade this approach was generally accepted and was chosen as the treatment for many disorders. However, the theoretical underpinnings of behaviour therapy did not keep up with its clinical development. To fill this gap, therapists became interested in the use of cognitive theory which rejected the concept that learning consisted merely of associations between stimuli and responses. Lang's (1993) 'three systems' approach was adopted widely because it seemed to be a useful alternative to the unitary behavioural view of psychological problems. His notion was that there are three relatively independent response systems: behavioural, cognitive/affective and physiological. Conceptualizing psychological problems from these different angles made it possible to link together a wide range of symptom patterns. Behavioural analysis was thus improved, which resulted in more comprehensive treatment approaches. The cognitive theorists emphasized the understanding and intellectual interpretation of experiences in the learning process. As learning occurs in organized patterns it is these patterns we learn, not the specific details of the tasks. It is necessary for a situation to be fully understood, taking into account the interrelationship of different factors or variables, before behaviour can be changed successfully. Therefore the learning of communication skills will be made easier by using cognitive concepts.

The term 'cognitive behaviour therapy' was first used in the scientific literature in the mid-1970s and by the end of the decade a number of controlled trials of this form of treatment had been published. In a relatively short period of time, cognitive behaviour therapy has established itself as one of the most promising avenues in psychotherapy. Clinical procedures are systematically delineated and their application with a wide range of client problems have been empirically tested.

Cognitive behavioural treatment approaches use the model of cognitive 'schemata', stable mental representations based on past experiences. These schemata are important for the manner in which we process information. Beck (1964) proposed that in depression the central schemata give rise to negative cognitions, for example, 'I will always be a failure' which are triggered by stressful events. In Beck's view dysfunctional schemata persist because clients employ erroneous logic. For example, they may overgeneralize from single instances, or focus selectively on negative features in a situation instead of balancing positive and negative aspects.

A further important development of cognitive behaviour theory was Bandura's (1977) analysis of self-regulatory processes. This was based on the idea that all voluntary behaviour change was mediated by clients' *perceptions* of their ability to perform the behaviour in question (self-efficacy).

Another cognitive approach which generated a great deal of interest among behavioural researchers was Meichenbaum's self-instruction training (1975). He suggested that behaviour change can be brought about by changing the instructions that clients' give themselves (internal dialogue), turning the maladaptive and upsetting thoughts to more constructive self-talk.

Beck's (1970, 1976) cognitive therapy and Ellis' (1962, 1996) rational emotive therapy (originally RET, now Rational Emotive Behaviour Therapy, REBT) were slowly adapted and these have progressed to probably being the most important of the cognitive approaches. Developed originally for the treatment of depression, Beck's cognitive therapy has now been extended to be applied to a wide range of emotional disorders. In both approaches the client is helped to recognize patterns of thinking which relate to dysfunctional behaviour. Systematic discussion and carefully structured behavioural assignments are used to help clients evaluate and modify both their dysfunctional thoughts and the consequent maladaptive behaviour.

Cognition and Social Skills

From a cognitive–social perspective, Ladd and Mize (1983) saw the following social skills as necessary for effective functioning:

1. Knowledge of specific interpersonal actions and how they fit into different kinds of person-to-person situations.
2. Ability to convert knowledge of social nuances into the skilled performance of social actions in various interactive contents.
3. The ability to evaluate accurately skilful and unskilful behaviour and to adjust one's behaviour accordingly.

The development of interactive skills involves not only the acquisition of certain rules but also being able to cope with contradictory rules of communication, e.g. being truthful versus being polite. In order to resolve such conflicts successfully a higher cognitive process is involved. A large number of skills are necessary in order to carry out the sophistic-ated interdependent interactions required in communication. These abilities would include:

1. Viewing one's own strengths and weaknesses realistically.
2. Recognizing and labelling one's own emotions in relation to external events.
3. Being empathic, i.e. being aware of the feelings of others, which would include the interpretation of verbal and non-verbal com-munication.

Bruch (1981) found that high-assertive college students showed signific-antly greater conceptual complexity (CC) than low-assertive subjects. Conceptual complexity is related to the rules or schemas that help discriminate, encode, and retrieve information concerning social cues. If the individual is able to process more complex situations, his ability to deal with interpersonal conflicts and resolve them positively is enhanced. Increased complexity allows the individual to discriminate situational cues more precisely, thus permitting broader and more varied viewpoints, to integrate information and to increase tolerance for conflict.

In an additional study, Bruch *et al.* (1981) directly investigated the rela-tionship between CC and assertive behaviour. They found that assertive behaviour of high and low CC subjects did not differ in simple situations but that in difficult ones, e.g. continuing relationships, the high CC subjects maintained assertive responses over a greater number of interac-tions. The authors noted that the abstract cognitive styles characteristic of high CC individuals are particularly important in complex social situations because such instances require multiple perspectives and flexibility. This is in contrast to simple situations, in which an appropriate response is directly indicated by social norms. Bruch *et al.* suggest that rather than focusing on specific cognitive interventions designed to alter irrational beliefs, low CC clients may benefit most from training which combines general problem solving skills and overt performance skills.

Social skills training is primarily geared towards the teaching of specific or complex behavioural skills. The cognitive approach progresses from a concrete level to a more abstract level and thus training focuses more on the process of interaction, e.g. problem solving. We know that 'self-efficacy' (Bandura, 1977) can be impaired by negative beliefs, unrealistic expectations or faulty attributions (the attempt to explain an event following its occurrence). Cognitive therapy addresses itself to these negative 'mind-sets'. Clients are assisted in understanding the emotions and behaviours which affect social interaction as well as exploring the consequences of their actions which may precipitate the need for change. They are encouraged to conceptualize themselves as the agents of their development, actively generating alternative strategies, making hypotheses regarding the consequences of these new behaviours and testing them. In this process self-monitoring, self-evaluation and self-reinforcement have important roles to play in both the acquisition and particularly the maintenance of new skills and behaviours.

Self-management Strategies: Self-monitoring, Stimulus Control, and Self-reward

Self-management is a process whereby the therapist explains to the client techniques he can apply to achieve a self-set goal. This could be modifying aspects of his environment, changing his self-talk and applying self-reinforcement.

Initially clients are often hesitant about using self-management techniques because they have expectations that the therapist will work things out for them rather than their doing it for themselves. Therefore it is necessary for the therapist to motivate clients actively to initiate change. When this is agreed, self-management procedures can help the client to develop his full potential. The first important technique in self-management is for the client to observe and record particular behaviours, thoughts, feelings, and actions about himself and the interaction with outside events. Virtually all forms of therapy encourage client 'self-exploration' or train the client to observe his behaviour and cognitions. This period of data collection allows therapists and clients to define the problem and to develop appropriate therapeutic strategies.

The following are the steps for a self-management programme:

1. The client identifies and records a problem behaviour, its antecedents and consequences. These baseline data have to be collected before any self-management strategies are used. *A teacher (Mrs. X) who has a voice problem (misuse of voice) reports that she has difficulty with her voice production when she is tired, anxious to keep control in the classroom, in a smoky atmosphere or when she shouts at her family.*
2. The desired behaviour is clearly identified (goal setting).
3. The therapist discusses possible self-management strategies: stimulus control — pre-arrangement of antecedents or cues to increase or decrease a target behaviour; and self-reward — a self-determined positive stimulus following a desired behaviour.

4. The client selects one or more strategies in an appropriate combination (some focusing on antecedents of behaviour, others on consequences).

5. After the client has agreed to a consistent use of these strategies they are demonstrated and practised during the session. *Mrs. X has agreed to look at how she might prevent herself from getting overtired. She suggests that she reorganizes her household duties so that she gets more help from her family. The therapist would then practise with Mrs X various ways of approaching each family member for their help.*

6. The client applies the strategies *in vivo* and records the frequency of use of each strategy and to what degree the client was able to realize the desired behaviour.

7. The client's data are reviewed and evaluated by the therapist and client. Depending on the results, the next steps are discussed, prepared, and put into practice (*in vivo*) by the client. The importance of self-reinforcement is repeatedly stressed.

Well-constructed and well-executed self-management programmes have the advantage that they increase a client's perceived control over his environment and decrease his dependence on therapy which, in turn, enhances the client's motivation for active involvement in therapy. A further advantage of self-management strategies is that they enable generalization of treatment effects. A major part of therapy is transferred into real-life settings.

A major challenge to any helper is finding ways to strengthen a client's commitment to using self-management strategies and a critical issue is the ability of the client to keep to the agreed 'contract'.

Self-instruction

Meichenbaum (1977) shares the view held by Luria (1961) and Vygotsky (1962) that much behaviour is guided by internal self-statements. As inner speech assumes a 'self-governing role', an alteration of self-statements would result in behavioural changes. Self-instructional training (Meichenbaum, 1977) teaches clients to be aware of their covert statements or 'thought processes' and alter them to change their behaviour. Five components are involved in this process:

1. The model engages in the target behaviour while speaking aloud the covert statements that guide the behaviour. This verbalizing of thought processes is called 'cognitive modelling'.

2. The client performs the target behaviour whilst the model verbally directs him by prompting the instructions that were modelled in the first step.

3. The client performs the behaviour whilst speaking aloud the instructions modelled previously.
4. The client whispers the instructions whilst engaging in the behaviour.
5. The client engages in the behaviour whilst guiding his activities via sub-vocal speech, i.e. thinking the instructions taught in the previous steps.

The sequence of self-instruction for children is the same as for adults but their linguistic level will need to be taken into consideration and instructions modelled appropriately. Training usually consists of four stages:

1. The behaviour to be changed is identified.
2. Instructions are given to focus attention on the task and guide behaviour to produce a solution.
3. Social reinforcement is provided as feedback to sustain appropriate behaviour.
4. Performance is evaluated and steps are taken to correct errors. It is then repeated, with instructions becoming more abbreviated and automatic.

Drawing on Meichenbaum's work, Kendall and Braswell (1985) suggest the following self-instructional statements for cognitive therapy with children:

1. Problem definition: "Let' see, what am I supposed to do?"
2. Problem approach: "I have to look at all the possibilities".
3. Focusing of attention: "I'd better concentrate and think only of what I am doing".
4. Choosing an answer: "I think it's this one".
5. Self-reinforcement: "Hey, not bad, I really did a good job".

or

6. Coping statement: "Oh, I made a mistake. Next time I'll try and go slower and concentrate more and maybe I'll get the answer right".

Here is an example of how a child can be taught to change his cognitive strategies which will bring about a more successful interaction:

> *Therapist:* You just started playing with a new toy. A boy comes over to you and says, "Give me that toy right now! I want to play with it". (Therapist holds up one finger), "What's the problem? . . . that boy wants me to give him my toy but I'm not finished playing with it". (Holds up two fingers), "What can I do? . . . well, I could

just yell at him and tell him 'no' . . . or I could just give him the toy
. . . or I could tell him that I'm using it and he can have it after I've
finished". (Holds up three fingers), "How would those work? . . .
if I yell at him and tell him 'No' I'll get to keep my toy but he
might get real mad and punch me . . . if I just give him the toy then
I won't get to finish playing with it . . . if I tell him that he can have
it when I've finished then I'll keep my toy until I am through and
then share it with him later . . . Yes, that last one is the best
choice". Therapist role plays the final response (holds up four
fingers), "How did I do? . . . I did a good job. I kept my toy until I
was finished and then shared it with the boy. I can also tell
because we both look happy, we are smiling and not yelling at
each other".

The child then goes through the same situation employing self-instruction. The therapist might use situation cards, each child/patient picking a
situation and going through the self-instruction procedure. Therapists
should encourage participants to discuss the statements they say to
themselves regarding what makes it harder or easier for them to be
assertive, and then model the appropriate self-statement.

This type of cognitive self-control training is important in the
successful acquisition, application and maintenance of social skills. It
assists the child/adult in shifting his locus of control from external to
internal; to see *himself* as the arbiter of change rather than attribute
his successes or failures to events and forces outside his control. The
child/adult who attributes his failures in interpersonal relationships to
events outside himself will be less likely to be motivated to make
personal changes. Glenwick and Jason (1984) suggest that children
who are able to make changes in their attributional style as a result of
cognitive self-control therapy have greater expectations of being
successful.

Cartledge and Milburn (1986) consider cognitive self-control techniques to be most appropriate for impulsive children who need to learn
to 'stop and think'. They see anxious inhibited reflective children as
profiting more from the cognitive restructuring approaches.

Shure and Spivack (1979) report that their programme, the interpersonal cognitive problem solving approach, could not only be applied to
relatively normal children but also that it has been used with 'varying
degrees of success' with 'learning-disabled children 6 to 12 years of age'.

To help children understand cognitive changes that they make in
their real world, a record sheet (see Figure 3.1) can be helpful in
collecting information.

Now that you have learned how to ignore teasing, you are ready to practise this at home as well as at school. Think about this for the next two days. Write down in the space below what happened when you ignored someone teasing you.

1. Describe the incident when you were teased.

_____

_____

_____

2. How did you ignore it?

_____

_____

_____

3. What did you say to yourself to help you ignore the teasing?

_____

_____

_____

4. What did the other person do?

_____

_____

_____

5. Did this solve the problem?

_____

_____

_____

6. How did you feel afterwards?

_____

_____

_____

Figure 3.1: Children's record sheet

Cognitive Restructuring

Cognitive restructuring is a technique that helps clients to cope with heightened emotional reactions and resist self-defeating social responses. It is aimed at helping the client identify faulty or self-defeating cognitions or perceptions and replace these with more constructive, self-enhancing views. The rationale for such treatment is that negative self-statements cause emotional distress, that the client's positive belief should be strengthened and that 'self-talk' can influence performance.

'Worrying' is probably one of the most debilitating of 'cognitive behaviours'. Therefore the reduction of worrying is at the centre of cognitive restructuring. The aim is to help the client to identify negative self-statements and then encourage him to generate positive coping statements in place of the negative ones. Beck (1963) used the term 'automatic thoughts' to describe those discrete specific thoughts that occur very rapidly, seemingly unprompted by events and which are not the result of voluntary thinking. After having educated the client about cognitive therapy, the first task is to identify these negative automatic thoughts which come 'out of the blue'. In most cases they are specific in content, providing interpretation of events and often include predictions about situations. They can occur with little awareness. These negative, automatic thoughts are perceived by the client as unchangeable facts or truths: 'The future only consists of problems. I never do anything right. Everything turns out badly.'

> *Example:*
> An adolescent who stutters and is depressed is unlikely to take the initiative in seeking a job. His thinking is likely to be dysfunctional: 'I'm useless, I won't get a job'. 'It's a waste of time trying'. 'Who will employ a stutterer?' By changing his cognitions or beliefs he is more likely to behave in a way that leads to success.

Once the client identifies his negative thoughts during problem situations, coping thoughts are developed by client and therapist and practised. Examples of coping self-statements might be: 'This task is a challenge, rather than a threat. I can work out a plan to cope with this. Concentrate on the task!'

As Beck *et al.* (1979) noted, clients rarely test the reality of their thoughts as they selectively attend to negative stress-increasing stimuli. The therapist will need to pursue clients' negative thoughts until such time as they are able to question their own beliefs and ideas. Once clients can look at their thoughts more objectively, and understand the effect of negative automatic thoughts on feelings and behaviours, they will then manage to distance themselves gradually from these unhelpful/negative cognitions. This process is supported by setting up personal experiments (homework) to practise new and constructive trains of thought in real-life situations.

Rational Emotive Behaviour Therapy (REBT)

REBT, as developed by Ellis (1975), holds that most problems are the result of 'irrational beliefs'. We label our 'emotional' reactions according to our conscious or unconscious evaluations, interpretations or philosophies. Ellis states that we feel anxious or depressed because we strongly convince ourselves that it is terrible when we fail at something or that we cannot stand the pain of being rejected. The basic ideas can be traced as far back as the Stoic philosopher, Epictetus, 2000 years ago, who wrote that there are virtually no legitimate reasons why human beings need to make themselves terribly upset or emotionally disturbed, no matter what kind of negative experiences they are confronted with. According to this school of thought we are 'free' to feel strong emotions, such as sorrow, regret, annoyance or determination to change social conditions. However, emotions like guilt, depression or anxiety are seen as self-defeating and inappropriate and should therefore be changed. Ellis (1975) compiled a list of 'irrational ideas' that, in his view, cause and sustain emotional disturbance: 'It is a dire necessity for an adult to be loved by everyone for everything he does'. 'It is horrible when things are not the way one would like them to be'. (Ellis, 1975, pp. 61 – 62).

REBT strives to resolve a client's problems by 'cognitive control of illogical emotional responses'. The client is re-educated through the use of what Ellis (1975) called the ABCDE Model. This model involves showing the client how irrational beliefs (B) about an activity or action (A) result in irrational or inappropriate emotional consequences (C). The client is then taught to dispute (D) the irrational beliefs, which are not based on facts and have no supporting evidence, and to then discern the effects (E). The effects should be a change in cognitions and in behaviour. Clients will need to develop the ability to 'dispute' their irrational beliefs and develop rational self-statements. When disputing the irrational beliefs the therapist uses a repertoire of questions like, 'Does the belief make you feel better?', 'Does it help you accomplish your goals?', 'Would everybody have the same belief in this situation?' *Counters* will be developed during therapy sessions: a counter is a thought which argues against another thought and includes thinking or behaviour in an opposite direction, hopefully convincing oneself of the falsity of a belief: 'I am worthless if I fail this test'. A directly opposite counter would be: 'My grade on this test has nothing to do with my worth as a person'.

Knaus (1974) developed a rational emotive therapy programme for children which includes these steps:

1. Helping children learn about feelings.
2. Challenging irrational beliefs, helping children recognize their irrational belief systems.
3. Challenging feelings of inferiority, helping children learn to evaluate themselves and others in positive terms.
4. Helping children become realistic about issues related to perfectionism.
5. Teaching children to think in terms of what they would like to have happen rather than irrational '*must* and *should* happen'.

In order to assist generalization of therapy effects into everyday life, the following additional techniques might be used.

Cognitive Rehearsal: Clients are instructed to imagine they are entering a social situation that they usually avoid. They are then asked to imagine the same situation whilst covertly repeating positive rational self-statements that have been developed during the 'disputing' process.

Distraction Methods: These can be used to control emotional reactions by redirecting attention away from the emotional experiences to specific aspects in the environment. Clients might distract themselves from their emotional reactions either by initiating relaxation procedures or by focusing their attention on an object that is present in the anxiety provoking situation and describing it to themselves in great detail.

Rational Emotive Imagery: This was designed to bridge the gap between 'intellectual' and 'emotional' insight (Maultsby and Ellis, 1974). Clients are encouraged to visualize the anteceding event (A) which is often the worst they can realistically imagine. Whilst keeping such an image clearly in mind, clients are encouraged to practise the new rational beliefs that have previously been identified through 'disputing'. Clients are encouraged to go over their rational belief in their imagination and are then asked to observe changes in their emotional reactions. They are encouraged to practise this technique several times a day, usually for several weeks.

Additional behavioural techniques used in therapy are modelling and role playing (see pages 43 and 46). All the techniques used in therapy sessions are a basis to be transferred to real life which is achieved through homework assignments. The tasks should be concrete, observable and measurable and they should increase in difficulty over the course of therapy.

Problem Solving

The problem solving technique is the most complex skill taught in social skills training. It enables patients to adopt a more constructive, rapid and effective way of dealing with difficult situations. Good problem solvers tend to show better social adjustment than those with limited skills (Spivack and Shure, 1974).

D'Zurilla (1988, p. 86) defines problem solving as a 'cognitive–affective–behavioural process through which an individual (or group) attempts to identify, discover, or invent effective means of coping with problems encountered in everyday living'. Problem solving is learning to work systematically through a set of steps for analysing a problem, discovering new approaches, evaluating these and developing strategies for implementing them in everyday life. The logic of problem solving is 'common sense'. The fact that the steps of problem solving are basically available to clients makes it easier to use them within therapy.

A productive way to begin the problem solving process is to ask clients what advice they would have for someone else who had a similar difficult experience. Or what advice might they offer themselves if they were in a better state of mind? These questions encourage clients to appreciate that they do have problem solving capabilities within their repertoires but that thoughts and feelings can inhibit or interfere with the process. Within a therapeutic context the term 'problem' refers to specific situations or sets of related situations to which one must respond in order to function effectively. The problems with which clients come to therapy are complex, not only because strong human feelings are often involved, but also because social settings and systems can play an important role in generating and sustaining problems. Because of this complexity, therapists not only need to understand and appreciate the difficulties and ramifications of a given problem but also they have to take care to avoid being overwhelmed by it; even in the face of chaos, they will need to be able to help the client do *something*. Since it is impossible to deal with all problems at once, it is necessary to focus on issues that seem to need immediate attention or seem to be common to a number of the client's problems or can be managed in view of available resources. As it is easier to deal with moderately difficult problems rather than serious emotional conflicts, therapists should encourage the solving of more simple difficulties regarding behaviour and situations in the early stages.

The initial analysis of the problem helps clients to choose or explore behaviours that seem important in terms of generating or maintaining a problem. When clients are helped to place their worries in perspective, they sometimes realize that the original problems are symptoms of more fundamental difficulties.

The stages of problem solving as developed by D'Zurilla (1986) are as follows.

Treatment Rationale: The rationale explains the purpose and gives an overview of the steps needed to strengthen a client's belief that problem solving is an important coping skill.

Problem Orientation: The therapist determines the individual problem solving style. Clients with maladaptive coping styles blame themselves or others for the problems. Maladaptive coping styles are characterized by minimizing the benefits of problem solving and maximizing or exaggerating the negative consequences that may occur from failure successfully to solve the problem. If necessary, the therapist uses cognitive techniques (for example cognitive restructuring) to overcome cognitive and emotional obstacles to problem solving. The client will need to fully understand and agree that time, energy and commitment are required to be able to solve problems successfully.

Problem Identification and Clarification: Problems cannot be dealt with if they remain vague and non-specific. They need to be identified in terms of specific experiences, behaviours, and feelings. During this stage the client is asked to gather as much objective information about the problem as possible. To obtain this information it is necessary to identify the obstacles that are creating difficulties or are preventing effective responses. Once the problems have been identified and defined, realistic goals are set. What would the client like to happen as a consequence of solving the problem? The goals should be realistic and attainable. It is important to identify the obstacles that might interfere with attaining the set goals. Finally, the therapist should help the client to understand that the complexities involved in most problem situations usually require the problem to be viewed from several different angles.

Generation of Different Solutions: At this stage of problem solving the client tries to generate as many alternative solutions to the problem as possible. The client should think of what he could do or ways to handle the problem. The client and therapist should let their imagination run free and think of a large variety of possibly new and original solutions, no matter how peculiar they might seem at first. Judgement or critical evaluation should be deferred. In the first instance, a large quantity of ideas is required and this will offer the client more choices which will improve the quality of his final choices.

• Aim for quantity not quality.
• Do not judge the ideas — their value can be assessed later.
• Let the mind wander — wild and quirky ideas can turn out to be winners.
• Build on ideas of others — expanding and adding to ideas already offered.

This 'brain-storming process' should carry on until client and therapist are satisfied that the ideas produced are a good basis for the next step.

Decision Making: The client is instructed to screen the list of available alternatives and eliminate solutions that are risky or not feasible. The outcomes for each remaining alternative are then considered. They should maximize benefits and minimize costs. Each solution is evaluated using these criteria:

- Will the problem be solved?
- How much time and effort will be needed to solve the problem?
- What effect will it have on overall personal and social well-being?

The client will need to look not only at the number of alternative solutions, but also at the quality and appropriateness of them. It may be that the problem cannot be solved with one of the existing solutions, therefore it might be necessary to collect more information or to redefine the problem. If the questions have been satisfactorily answered, the client is ready to implement the solution.

Solution Implementation and Verification: The chosen solutions should then be tested out in order to verify that they can solve the problem. However, it is possible that the client is unable to implement the chosen solutions because of behavioural deficits, or because they evoke strong emotions or negative cognitions. In this event the therapist will be required to use other clinical techniques such as self-management, self-monitoring, correct evaluation and reinforcement.

If the solutions prove to be unsuccessful the problem solving strategy will need to be recycled.

Many speech and language impaired patients have great difficulty problem solving and therapists will need to take into account the degree of intellectual and physical of handicap of the client and to simplify their instructions and expectations accordingly.

Example:
Problem: Client is unable to maintain eye contact.
Suggested solutions:

1. Ask someone to remind me when I am looking away.
2. Do an exercise on observation.
3. Ask someone to look away so that I feel uncomfortable.
4. Ask the person to whom I am talking to close his eyes and I will touch him on his arm when I am ready to look.
5. Wear dark glasses.
6. When I look at my conversation partner, he or she is to smile and nod.
7. I am to smile and nod when my partner gives me good eye contact.
8. Instruct myself to give eye contact every 5 seconds.

Selected solutions in order of preference: First choice 1, then 6, 7, 2.

It might be necessary to the speech and language impaired client to offer a series of suggestions in a visual form, i.e. picture sequences or gesture.

Problem solving and cognitive techniques in general enable clients to take personal responsibility for exploring and modifying their attitudes and self-concepts. This self-attributed change will enable the client not only to overcome current problems better but also to develop the skills necessary to cope with similar ones in the future, thus avoiding relapse.

Chapter 4
Principles and Elements of Training

Introduction

The most important aspect of psychotherapy is the client/therapist relationship. It is generally accepted that the Rogerian therapeutic variables 'warmth, empathy and positive regard' are necessary but not sufficient for a positive outcome in therapy. Behavioural social skills training adds some elements which have been developed to give concrete and practical help in achieving therapy goals. Optimally, the social skills therapist should personally have a wide repertoire of interpersonal skills from which he can draw therapeutic interventions. Therapists should structure the process by explaining their role, informing clients about the necessary steps and what is to be expected from them. Geared to the particular client's level of sophistication, a thorough rationale for the intervention is presented. This should help to demystify the treatment process and underscore the fact that the client is fully capable of initiating and maintaining the steps necessary for self-improvement with only limited support from the therapist. The training approach of social skills training (SST) stands in contrast to other therapies that concentrate on changing underlying 'neurotic defences and conflicts'.

SST rests on the assumption that people act purposefully, that they are sensitive to the effects of their behaviour and that they 'learn' insofar as they take steps to modify their behaviour in the light of past experience. SST should be designed to enhance this process by developing better observational, performance, and cognitive skills. Deficiencies might involve inappropriate goals, inaccurate perception or translation (coding, decoding information) or deficient performance. Other factors might be important as well, such as anxiety in social situations.

In communication skills training, the therapist is a teacher and the client a student. The client's problems are viewed as deficits of competency rather than as abnormalities of illness. The medical sequence, illness → diagnosis → prescription → therapy → cure becomes client dissatisfaction (or ambition) → goal setting → goal teaching → goal achievement. The view of clients' problems as skills deficits is the basis for the educational model of communication skills training. By defining clients' problems as skill deficits and presenting the tools to correct these deficits, the therapist encourages clients to take charge not only of their own treatment but also of some aspects of their own lives as well. Clients who are taught problem solving skills are able to solve many diverse problems rather than working through one problem with a therapist which they would be unlikely to generalize to other areas. An overview of the process of treatment is shown in Table 4.1.

Table 4.1. Social skills training: Overview of the process of treatment

Goals	Techniques
Establish therapeutic alliance, Assess social performance and perception skills. Define goals, establish treatment contract.	Empathy and rapport. Interview. Observation, paper-and-pencil tests.
Plan and implement teaching activities — provide alternative responses to undesirable behaviours.	Instruction, modellling, role play, feedback, homework.
Transfer and maintenance. Improving the support system: Increased understanding of handicap and patient's needs by family or carers.	Counselling.
Reintegration into original environment if possible, strengthening of familial relationship.	Counselling, encouragement/ reinforcement.

The teaching/learning methods of communication skills training derive from education and psychology. From the field of education comes structured discussion, simulation and game playing. The field of psychology has provided the principles of social-learning theory, in particular, transfer of training, observational learning techniques such as modelling and self-confrontation, behavioural rehearsal and feedback (cueing or reinforcement). Brief introductory texts, or role instructions and audio and video technologies are also used.

These teaching/learning methods are characterized by:

1. Active participation of clients in the learning process.
2. Focus on specific behaviours (internal and external) which are learned and maintained (tasks are presented from simple to complex).

3. The programmes are based on established learning principles of modelling, observing, discriminating, reinforcing, and generalizing.
4. The training includes both didactic and experiential elements.
5. The courses are highly structured (systematic presentation of material).
6. Goals are clear.
7. Progress is monitored.

Learning takes place on different levels: behaviour (specific actions), skills and capabilities (what can be done), beliefs and values (what are the things that matter) and to a lesser degree on the level of identity (basic sense of self, core values).

Defining operational goals is one of the mainstays of behaviour therapy in general and social skills training in particular. Yet in order to do this, we need a clear concept of socially appropriate and inappropriate behaviour. How should social inadequacy be defined or measured? Adequate social behaviour will be judged against social norms and consequently it suffers from the inevitable difficulties of being vague, because social norms differ between social subgroups and because of the subjectivity of assessing certain behaviour. Appropriate social patterns vary with age, sex, social class, etc. Therapists have to be sensitive to this and have to strive to develop goals with clients which are acceptable in their environment/culture. Still, there are some basic rules which can be generalized beyond cultural 'restraints'. Showing little variation in facial expression during communication, looking predominantly blank and unsmiling, keeping a closed posture, being inflexible, and not looking at the other person would generally be deemed unacceptable.

During the first stage of training, clients are presented with an analysis of the skill. The therapist might give a short lecture, show a video or use handouts. The use of videos facilitates skill discrimination and enables participants to appreciate the central aspects which are involved in this specific skill. In the next stage clients have the opportunity to practise this skill within the group. This is followed by feedback, where participants are made aware of what they did during practice in relation to what they were trying to achieve and what effects this had on their practice partners. It is important that clients attribute to themselves any change which occurs. Therapists may encourage this 'self-attribution', not only by conceptualizing the course as an educational, skill-training process, but also by encouraging clients to analyse in detail how *they* brought about the changes. This will enable clients to be in a better position to use the developed coping strategies in the future, building on their own experience.

Skills training progresses from simple to more intricate, and learning a new skill involves learning subskills. During the period of skill acquisition these subskills are not integrated and the learner is self-conscious and awkward. Only with time and practice, which should be provided within the group, will the components require less and less conscious attention, allowing the client to devote increasing attention to more sophisticated strategies. It is important to give sufficient time for practice and application within the safety of the group, to enable a fair standard to be reached, thereby increasing the likelihood of successful generalization. Communication skills therapists should have a working knowledge of the competencies people need to master life challenges such as resolving a crisis or developing a relationship. There are clear guidelines associated with the learning of a skill. Therefore we would expect that training clients in the use of various communication skills will be a relatively straightforward procedure. None the less, there are a number of possible pitfalls one might encounter. Some of the more common problems will briefly be reviewed here.

1. Clients frequently enter therapy with the idea that something will be done *to* them or *for* them. The idea that they are provided with an occasion for learning general skills in dealing with their specific problems is initially quite alien. Therefore clients have to be given an appropriate rationale for their training procedure, 'socializing' clients as quickly as possible into a coping skills orientation.
2. The change process in most cases is gradual. Clients often find it difficult to see the progress they are making and as a result may become discouraged. Therapists should increase clients' awareness of the changes by encouraging them to self-monitor their success at coping with various communicative situations and then compare this with how they responded (or might have responded) to similar situations prior to the training. Self-reinforcement for progress should be encouraged.
3. The maintenance of change over time is very relevant to the training process. Problem solving training which deals with regression or relapse should be emphasized to help stabilize gains. Overlearning responses to difficult situations (social pressure, negative emotional states) should reduce the risk of regression. We all know that having a coping skill in one's repertoire does not ensure that it will be used. We might be most proficient in helping others place upsetting situations into a more reasonable perspective, but when we are confronted with upsetting events ourselves, we do not use such coping skills properly. Developing an individually appropriate signal or cue for coping might help in this respect. Therapists should help clients find the most effective way of getting 'in touch' with their feelings as a trigger for an appropriate reaction.

If relapse occurs, it is important that it is dealt with in a constructive way. The slip should not be seen as evidence of inadequate personal efficacy as this view can undermine subsequent coping efforts because the inference is made that the client is not really capable of handling stresses. Therapists should encourage clients to anticipate failures and setbacks and discuss in great detail how they should respond to such lapses. Actual failures that happen during the course of therapy might be used to develop appropriate coping responses and establish a sense of self-efficacy despite these difficulties. The discussion of relapse should be done in a sensitive manner. Therapists do not wish to convey the expectancy that training will lead to failure, but on the other hand, it should be pointed out that it would be unrealistic to assume that therapy would lead to an effective handling of *any* difficult situation.

4. In the past the topic of 'resistance' was relatively untouched in the behaviour therapy literature. This has changed and therapists are encouraged to be sensitive to and actively solicit evidence of disagreement, non-compliance and other uncooperative behaviours on the part of the client. Therapists should be aware of non-verbal signals of negative reactions. If she notices them, she should comment on them, encouraging the client to discuss these freely, as they are a valuable source of information guiding the treatment process. It might be useful to warn clients in the beginning about potentially inconvenient or troublesome aspects of homework and other therapeutic assignments, as this can increase compliance. If therapists encounter resistance, they should not try to break it and start a power struggle, but they should discuss the problem and if they are unable to gain the client's cooperation for a specific assignment, they should modify the actual treatment approach.

Modelling

Modelling is a demonstration by a therapist or group member of how a situation may be managed in a more effective way. Showing a person what to do can often be more productive than just telling him. Non-verbal as well as verbal behaviours can be demonstrated and attention drawn to those of importance.

When working with groups, using other group members who can exhibit the desired behaviour as models can be very helpful. Modelling stimulates the learning of new skills and behaviours and exposes the learner to a range of skills not previously known or practised. Thus 'good behaviour' can be enhanced whilst undesirable behaviour can be reduced. It is necessary to give clear instructions identifying specific behaviours. Therapists will appreciate that clients may not be able to carry out any given modelled behaviour the first time. A combination of practice coupled with feedback will be necessary and it should be remembered that each person brings something of themselves to each behaviour, which will make it subtly different from the actual model.

Prompting

Prompting is the way in which an individual is directed how to behave. It can be done verbally by giving clear instructions, gesturally by giving hand signals, or physically by actually touching the person and guiding their body towards the desired behaviour. Authoritative prompts are helpful in spurring to action individuals who are reluctant to do or say anything. Even the most withdrawn and inhibited person will respond by complying with a prompt, provided that the goal is a small and simple piece of verbal or non-verbal behaviour.

Shaping

Shaping is the technique of starting from where the individual is at the present moment and rewarding small improvements in behaviour that gradually build up into the goal behaviour. There are several component parts of both verbal and non-verbal social interaction; each component is successfully trained until the total picture is satisfactorily expressed.

In Vivo Practice

In vivo practice is the generalization of therapy from the clinical situation to real life. It allows clients the opportunity to put into practice the skills they wish to improve. Generally, clients are trained in the therapy session to a degree that will enable them to practise the required skills outside therapy. However, sometimes the therapist will need to accompany certain clients on their *in vivo* practice until they are confident enough to carry out the skill on their own.

Positive Feedback (Reinforcement)

In order to help people change their behaviour they will need a great deal of positive feedback/reinforcement. The beneficial effect is greatest when praise is given during and immediately after the behavioural rehearsal or task. This can be in the form of verbal approval, applause or pats on the back — or all three! Each time someone takes part in any game, exercise or role play the therapist has an opportunity to strengthen desirable behaviour with praise. There cannot ever be too much!

Video Recording

This has become a most popular method of providing feedback in the training of communication skills and can speed up the therapy process as it enables clients to watch a replay of their behaviour and assess it in detail before trying again. Before working with clients using the video system, it is important that therapists have a signed agreement from them that they are willing to be videotaped. An assurance will need to be given as to what will happen to the video tapes on the cessation of treatment.

The therapist will need to consider how best to expose clients, whether adults or children, to being recorded on video as people react differently to the prospect of seeing themselves on film. Some children relish the opportunity whilst others have serious concerns. Older clients or those who have neurological disorders will be more apprehensive and fearful and the therapist will need to take this into consideration. Some people prefer to be recorded in the group for the first time so that no one person feels too exposed individually or responsible for sustaining the interaction.

When clients are viewing their behaviour on a video the therapist should first encourage them to make a positive statement about the recording before any criticism is made. All criticism should be made in a positive way. For example, Mrs. X had a voice problem and when she had difficulties she dropped her eye gaze and became very fidgety. When she observed herself doing this on the video recording the first thing she said was, 'Oh dear, how awful', and the therapist said, 'Wait a moment, let's talk about the things that were good'.

Homework Assignments

Very little progress from the clinical setting to real life will take place without practice. Therefore homework assignments are of prime importance. Clients, whether seen individually or as a group, should be given clearly specified tasks to perform between therapy sessions. These should relate to work carried out in the session or work that has been rehearsed. Homework should be positive, functional and related to behaviours that are naturally appropriate in the client's daily life, starting with specific skills and progressing to the integration of several skills to match normal behaviour. Homework can be group or individually based. The tasks should be recorded on a homework sheet or in a diary, and might contain the following questions:

- What skill will you use?
- What are the steps for the skill?
- Where will you try the skill?
- With whom will you try the skill?

Following the assignment, the report sheet should be completed:

- What happened when you did the homework?
- Which steps did you really follow?

- How well did you do the skill (excellent, good, fair, poor)?
- What do you think should be your next homework assignment?

Each session should commence with a report back on the assignments and positive feedback should be given. Homework will need to be adjusted for each client's skills and performance. If negative reactions occur during homework practice the client should be given a variety of options including positive self-instruction (see page 28) and further training where necessary.

Role Rehearsal

Role rehearsal is a core component of social skills training. It enables the client to enact brief scenes that simulate realistic situations. Emphasis is placed on the client's set goals regarding verbal and non-verbal behaviour. Every rehearsal is followed by positive feedback from the therapist and then constructive comments can be made as to how the individual might improve. The use of video in role rehearsal is extremely helpful as individuals can observe how they are making progress and set their own goals for improvement.

> *Example:* An adult stutterer has difficulty maintaining eye contact when engaged in conversation with a shop assistant. Having worked on improving his eye contact within the client/therapist interaction, he is now ready to engage in role rehearsal. The therapist should devise a contrived scenario where she or a group member will be a shop assistant and the stutterer will enter the shop and ask for his requirements with specific attention to his eye contact. Scenes can be varied and changed as necessary. It might be helpful to allow the stutterer to be the shop assistant while the therapist or other group member acts out a stutterer not giving adequate eye contact.

When the practice has reached a satisfactory level, the patient should have the opportunity to try out this behaviour *in vivo*, preferably accompanied by the therapist who can (a) support him and (b) observe any problems for later discussion and, if necessary, further role rehearsal.

Role Play

This teaching method has been used extensively in social skills training and is a dramatic process that involves several components. Although role play is an exercise that can be time-consuming and requires a high level of concentration from both therapist and participants, it is highly effective in bringing about changes in behaviour.

The rationale is to create a real-life social encounter in miniature and in an artificial way, for the purpose of analysing the situation, assessing the performance of various participants, and giving individual feedback with which they can improve their social interaction. Although many people are initially reluctant to participate in role play, they can become extremely adept, particularly when asked to help other people enact their problem. Corsini (1966, p. 9) defines role play most succinctly:

1. *It is a close representation of real-life behaviour.* Although staged, every effort is made to reconstruct the natural conditions as closely as possible. The situations enacted are ones which the participant has either previously encountered or will very likely experience in the near future.
2. *It involves the individual holistically.* That is, the participant is required to respond totally to the situation. In role playing the participant must think or employ cognitions, he must respond emotionally or use feeling, and he must act or use drama.
3. *It presents observers with a picture of how the client operates in real-life situations.* This aspect provides assessment information so that the observer can determine skill competence under various social conditions.
4. *Because it is dramatic, it focuses attention on the problem.*
5. *It permits the individual to see himself while in action in a neutral situation.* Role playing provides a mechanism whereby the individual may analyze his own behaviour and recognise how certain actions can trigger various responses (sometimes negative ones) from others.

In setting up the role play, the following facts of the situation should be established:

• Who is involved: the age, role and attitude of the participants including relevant facial expression and posture.
• Location of incident: the overall setting including all details, e.g. doors, windows, furniture.
• Timing of incident: time of day and date, weather and season, if relevant.
• The sequence of events.

The therapist should then assist the client in the choice of group members to enact the various roles. The following training methods can be used during the role play:

• Modelling: the desired behaviour may be modelled by a peer or the therapist and it is helpful for the client to be able to identify with the model.

- Prompting and shaping: the therapist should direct the role play giving clear verbal instructions, including hand signals when necessary, physically guiding the client towards the desired behaviour. It is important to build on the client's existing skills and gradually, with positive reinforcement, to progress towards the target behaviour.
- Positive feedback and reinforcement: this is an extremely important aspect of role play. Immediately following the exercise a positive statement should be made regarding a correct behaviour, before suggesting improvement. Feedback should be sought from the group as well as from the client.
- Video: This can be an extremely effective training aid.

Role Reversal

The essential feature of this technique is that the therapist and client can switch roles. This can be a very effective way of developing self-awareness, changing attitudes and encouraging empathic understanding.

> *Example:* The father of an adolescent stutterer was extremely upset because he did not like his son's long hair and was continually shouting at him to change it. Placing the father in the son's shoes with the therapist becoming the father, he was able to work out a more successful way of communicating with his son because he realized how angry he became when the 'father' spoke so badly to him.

At the end of role play, role rehearsal and role reversal, each participant should be 'de-roled' by the therapist requesting each member to state his real name and status.

Sculpting

Sculpting enables events, feelings and problems to be represented in a visual manner, which is particularly helpful for clients who have difficulty expressing themselves verbally. The complexity of the sculpting exercise can be varied according to needs. The following example illustrates a simple, direct use of sculpting:

> Adolescents are helped to explore their feelings and attitudes to their school by asking them to place themselves in relation to a chair which represents their school. A discussion of the significance of their placement would follow.

Sculpting is also an alternative to other problem solving methods and the following steps are involved:

1. The client's problem is identified.
2. He describes who is involved and the physical setting.
3. The client chooses members of the group to represent those persons who are part of the problem and places them in positions to reflect their respective relationships. Physical props might be used. If the client is not satisfied with the result he moves the members around until the different aspects of his problems are well represented.

   Example: George, aged 15 years, reports constant discord with his brother. He arranges his sculpt in the following way using group members. His mother and brother sit opposite and close to each other on the floor — this would indicate that they are in alliance. His father is placed on a chair looking away from the family setting, thus demonstrating a lack of involvement in family issues. George places himself in a standing position away from the family group looking towards the mother and brother. This would indicate his unhappy feelings regarding the closeness of his mother and brother from which he feels excluded.

4. When the sculpt has been arranged the client approaches each participant and introduces them to the group by 'doubling', i.e. placing his hand on their shoulder and taking their place.

   Example: George would place his hand on his brother's shoulder and say, 'I am John Brown; I am the eldest son; I am 17 years old; tall, good looking, sporty. I have a good time and get on well with Mum. I think George is moody and unhappy'.

Thus, the group members have a better understanding of the elements of the problem and the client could begin to gain insight into the feelings of the other people involved in his problem.

5. Each participant is then asked how they feel in their current position.
6. The client is instructed to rearrange the sculpt in a way that may resolve the problem. Various contributions may be tried and after each change participants should report how they feel about the change.
7. It is possible for participants to offer to make changes in the sculpt as well as the therapist, if appropriate.
8. The final sculpt should be a solution to the problem.
9. All participants should be de-roled by stating their own name and status.
10. After the completion of the sculpting exercise, a full discussion regarding the problem and solution should take place. This should help the client consider changes that need to be made.

Relaxation

Introduction

Relaxation training is widely used in the treatment of speech and language disorders because the physiological state of relaxation is incompatible with feelings of fear, anger and anxiety.

It can become an effective technique for reducing anxiety and coping with stress in general as it helps clients manage a wide variety of anxiety-provoking events. Acquiring a range of relaxation skills enables clients to become more aware of the bodily cues associated with anxiety and at the same time provides them with the means for reducing feelings of tension. Relaxation training can focus on both physical and mental relaxation and all methods can be equally effective. Clients should be encouraged to experiment with several types and to use the one that is best suited to their personal needs.

Both children and adults benefit from relaxation techniques as a decrease in anxiety levels allows them to manage themselves and their communication problem more effectively.

It is important that the client understands the concept of relaxation and this should be carefully explained before relaxation *per se* is taught. Instructions to clients will depend on their comprehension and physical skills and should be adapted accordingly. It is helpful to use the client's own words to describe a relaxed state, e.g. calm, easy. This is of particular significance with respect to younger children or clients with a limited vocabulary. Games that involve contrasting states of tension and relaxation can be used, such as robots (p. 217), tin soldiers and rag dolls (p. 160), stiff and wobbly foods (p. 161). This helps clients experience the feelings in an activity and can be brought to a cognitive level, using brainstorming to identify the children's own words to describe their experience of being a robot or rag doll. Therapists should then use these words when teaching any relaxation techniques.

Relaxation training should take place in a quiet environment, and bright lights should be avoided. The tone of voice and the rate of speech of the instructor are important. The voice should be calm, slightly monotonous, and the rate of talking smooth and slow.

Training Techniques

Progressive Relaxation. Jacobson (1938) introduced a relaxation technique in which clients are taught by alternately tensing and relaxing groups of muscles and being aware of the differences between the sensation of tension and relaxation. Progressive muscle relaxation can lead to deep levels of physical and mental relaxation. Clients are required to tense and relax the muscles in the forehead, eyes, jaws, neck, shoulders, upper back, biceps, forearms, hands, abdomen, groin, legs, hips, thighs, buttocks, calves and feet. Each muscle group is tensed for 5 seconds and then relaxed for 10 to 15 seconds. Progressively they are taught to relax those muscles without initial tensing and once they are capable of becoming relaxed on their own within a very short period of time, clients are in the position to use their relaxation skills to cope actively with anxiety-provoking situations. This method of training has been adapted for a variety of client groups, particularly for those with voice disorders, both functional and organic, in adolescent and adult stutterers, and in other clients who are able to lie on their backs without discomfort or sit in a large comfortable chair. It is common for clients to feel ill at ease during the first relaxation session but they should be encouraged to persevere. In order to enhance the client's practice session at home, the therapist should tape record the instructions on to a cassette for home practice.

Cue-controlled relaxation. Cue-controlled relaxation is aimed at enabling the client to achieve a state of relaxation in response to a verbal cue. Initially, deep muscle relaxation is taught, then the relaxed state is repeatedly associated with the cue word such as 'relax' or 'calm'. Whilst the client is deeply relaxed the therapist repeats the chosen cue word, e.g. 'relax' in time with the client's exhalation. After some practice the client should then repeat the cue word to himself without the therapist. Once the association is firmly established, the client should be able to use the chosen cue word to reduce anxiety in everyday situations.

Autogenic Training. Johannes Schultz (1969), a Berlin neurologist, developed the autogenic training method. The client is taught to instruct himself how to make his limbs heavy and warm:

> You are gradually going to become aware that your right leg is becoming heavy, as limbs do when they are thoroughly relaxed. In order to let it happen, say to yourself, 'my right leg is becoming heavy'. Repeat this slowly to yourself 10 times over a period of one minute. This induces the 'switching off' of that part of the motor area in the brain that controls the legs. The leg now 'realizes' that movement is not needed at present. If it is not getting heavy, repeat it for another minute or two. Then when it is feeling heavier than your left leg, say to yourself, 'my right leg is getting very warm', in exactly the same way for the same length of time. Now do the same with the left leg.

These instructions are then applied to other parts of the body.

Physiological Relaxation. Mitchell (1977) devised a relaxation regime which is physiologically based and caters for the normal as well as the physically handicapped population. The philosophy of her method is that conscious awareness of states of tension is provided by feedback from joints and skin, not muscles and tendons. Therefore, conscious relaxation is brought about by adjusting body posture. The instructions are simple and clear and can easily be adapted for children, using their own words, as previously described.

Controlled Breathing. When people are anxious or tense their breathing patterns often become shallow and irregular. This can cause an imbalance in levels of oxygen and carbon dioxide within the body which can in turn trigger the physical symptoms of anxiety. Greenberger and Padesky (1995) suggest that it is important to practise controlled breathing for at least four minutes, because this is roughly how long it takes to restore the balance of oxygen and carbon dioxide. The balancing works most effectively by breathing in and out for equal amounts of time. One hand should be placed on the upper chest and one on the stomach, the hand on the stomach should move out as breath is taken in. It is recommended that clients should breathe in to a slow count of four and out to a further slow count of four, for four minutes. They should breathe gently either through their mouth or nose.

Imagery. Many clients, including children, find the use of images helpful in deepening their experience of relaxation. These images can be real or fantasy, as it is the associated feelings of relaxation and calm that are more important than the image. It involves clients in actively visualizing scenes that they may find calming, peaceful and relaxing. Where therapists are guiding this visualization, it is useful to elicit the scenes and images from the clients to ensure that they are meaningful and relevant to the indi-viduals or group concerned. Children for example find images connected to lying in bed, the bath or floating in a swimming pool more relaxing than scenes associated with activity and excitement.

It is important to incorporate as many other senses as possible into the visual image. These may include smells, sounds and tactile sensations.

> Imagine you are walking along the beach, you may become aware of the sounds of the sea and seagulls, the smell of the sea, perhaps you can feel a gentle breeze and the warm sun on your skin.

In this way each one of the senses can contribute to the client's experi-ence of relaxation.

Practice plays an important role in the acquisition of any skill, including relaxation. The more the client practises the chosen relaxation technique the greater the development of the skill.

Distraction. Clients tend to focus on physical sensations and sometimes irrational thoughts when they become anxious. Distraction focuses attention away from the sensations and thoughts that contribute to the state of anxiety. By becoming absorbed in other activities or thinking, the cognitive fuel for anxiety will be shut off. This will in turn decrease or eliminate the anxiety symptoms. The more the client is able to absorb himself in other thoughts or activities, the more the anxiety will dissipate. Distraction will need to be practised for at least four minutes before noting a decrease in anxiety.

Generalization of Social Skills

Current literature offers little on the subject of generalization of social skills. However, in order for social skills training to be of worth, clients will need to demonstrate that they are able to adapt the skills taught into their everyday life in a variety of settings. It should follow that improvement in social interaction should carry over into untaught skills, i.e. a specifically trained skill will lead to the development of an untrained skill.

Clinical and research experience has shown that generalization does not necessarily occur in education and therapy programmes. Cooke and Apolloni (1976) demonstrated that when socially deficient children were integrated with normal students, they did not automatically improve their social interaction. Strain and Timm (1974) noted that behaviourally disordered children were often ignored by their peers, rather than becoming involved in interactions that facilitated the development of appropriate social behaviours. These examples indicate that training must take into account the client's environment outside the clinical setting and should address not only the improvement of performance in specific skills but also support the acquisition of a variety of strategies.

The long-term generalization of behavioural techniques such as modelling and practice might be improved by training participants in 'dissecting' social behaviour, i.e. increasing their ability to analyse important determinants in situations. Clients develop a better understanding of their behaviour, i.e. strategy, as well as plans and underlying tactics.

The transfer of skills will also be enhanced if trainers strive for maximum 'stimulus variability', thus training should incorporate a variety of partners, models and a wide array of role play situations.

An important feature of generalization is the use of homework practice from the outset of treatment. Homework assignments are carried out in the real world and indicate to the therapist how well clients are able to generalize their newly acquired skills.

When treating cases of severe mental or physical disability, therapists and carers will need to agree on modest aims regarding social interaction but nevertheless they will require an understanding of the strategies in order for any improvement to be maintained.

No behaviour will transfer and be maintained if it is not reinforced outside therapy. Therapists should have a complete understanding of the client's social background and normally it will be advisable to include the family, teachers and peers in a discussion of how the newly acquired skills can be reinforced outside the clinical setting. This reinforcement should not be indiscriminate but must be supplemented by corrective feedback. It might even be possible to incorporate family and peers into the training process according to the specific needs of the different client groups. The *primary* motivating factor for young children is their parents, whereas adolescents are more influenced by their peers. These primary social reinforcers should be considered according to the level of development in order to enhance generalization. Rustin (1987) has shown that the integration of the family into treatment leads to good therapeutic results. She developed a programme for the management of the stuttering child (incorporating social skills training) where parents and child work together to achieve and maintain fluency.

In summary, we list the factors that promote generalization, as detailed by Stokes and Baer (1977).

- Teach behaviours that will be supported by the natural environment. If the new repertoire of behaviours is reinforced outside therapy, the likelihood of it being maintained increases considerably.
- A variety of different response forms for each social skill should be taught in order to make clients more responsive to different cultural or ethnic backgrounds: having learned various responses, there should be an increase in flexibility during novel situations.
- A variety of stimulus situations should be included in order to help clients to initiate some of their own problem situations.
- Training should extend across different persons and settings, possibly some of them belonging to the natural environment. Peers can be incorporated in different ways, such as using group reinforcement strategies, using peer models and allowing peers to initiate social interactions.
- Fade training consequences: reinforcement should gradually fade from a continuous to intermittent schedules and finally, use delayed reinforcement.
- Train accurate self-reports of performance: when doing homework, clients should be able to report back precisely what they achieved and how they did it, as only this kind of self-control will enable them to develop their skills further.
- In order to train complex skills, structures and strategies rather than single and simple techniques, participants should be encouraged constantly to explore possible new responses that are potentially more effective and useful for their specific social environment.

- Training in general should be geared towards the development and enhancement of problem-solving skills, to yield more durable and broad intervention effects.

Table 4.2: Processes of Social Learning

Definition of social skill goal/Introduction to training unit		
Modelling	Modelling stimuli should be	• distinct • relevant • simple (to match the observer's abilities)
Attention/retention	Effectiveness of training is is increased, if	• model is reinforced for engaging in desired behaviour • modelling scene is brief and to the point • adapted to the level of intellectual functioning of observers
Behavioural rehearsal (Motor reproduction) (Training of skills)	Ability to reproduce depends on	• physical capabilities • past learning history (availability of specific responses necessary for task)
Feedback/ motivation (Contingent reinforcement for behaviour	Learning will be enhanced by	• accurate self-observation/ self-reinforcement • vicarious external reinforcement
Transfer of training	Transfer and maintenance are improved if	• training situation and reality are similar • overlearning takes place (training beyond first accurate reproduction of modelled behaviour) • conducted in natural environment *in vivo* exercises homework exercises
Long-term maintenance	Booster sessions	• attitude change if behaviour is consistently effective

Chapter 5
Group therapy

Setting up a Group

Therapy in groups has been established as a highly beneficial way of managing speech and language impaired clients. A great deal of our day-to-day social interactions are experienced in groups, therefore it seems logical that this format should lend itself well to the teaching of social and communication skills. It is important for therapists to structure the groups in a way that allows for easy generalization, e.g. that group training incorporates problems that are relevant to the daily life of participants. There are a large number of potential advantages for groups.

- Changes of attitudes, feelings and behaviour can occur through social interaction, through role modelling, reinforcement and feedback.
- Every group member is a potential helper as each has many strengths and resources as well as his own particular problems.
- The group setting is particularly suitable for those clients who find the intensity and intimacy of a one-to-one relationship in therapy too threatening.
- Group work in general is more economical of therapists' time and effort.

However, there are disadvantages to group work.

- Confidentiality is more difficult to maintain.
- Groups require specific resources, e.g. larger accommodation.
- The individual receives less attention.
- Group membership can increase stigma.
- Groups can be difficult to plan, organize and implement.

Every therapeutic approach has undesirable side-effects for some clients, therefore one has to consider this when assessing potential participants for groups.

Running a Group

The development of a group of individuals into a supportive helping unit is not an instant process, it takes time. To achieve this, the group leader helps members of the group to organize themselves, pool resources and set the stage for co-operative action. The time limit necessitates that the therapist is active in creating a structured format that enables each member to engage in significant interpersonal learning in every session. The appropriate balance between affect and cognition, and between task orientation (reason/logic) and process (dynamics) of communication is important. Process covers the social emotional aspects of group communication, feelings and attitudes of group members and how they relate to one another. Non-verbal communication plays a major role in this second dimension and therapists have to be aware of this element.

To analyse group communication Bales (1950) developed a system known as interaction process analysis. It contains 12 categories, six of which are concerned with task functions: giving opinions, giving evaluations, asking for or giving information, giving repetition or clarification, and asking for or giving suggestions or directions.

Six categories are related to positive or negative socio-emotional reactions: showing solidarity, helping or rewarding, showing tension release or satisfaction, showing agreement, acceptance, understanding, antagonism, and tension, withdrawing or asking for help, disagreeing or rejecting. In order to obtain a deeper understanding of the current stage a group is in, it might be useful to rate group interaction with these categories (possibly done by the group's co-leader). A more recent and more simple system developed by Honey (1988) was: seeking ideas, proposing, building, disagreeing, supporting, seeking clarification, clarifying/explaining/informing, and difficulty stating.

Tuckman (1965) noted that every group passes through four stages in its development. He described these as (1) forming, (2) storming, (3) norming, and (4) performing.

During the forming stage, members of the group are meeting for the first time and are usually on their 'best behaviour', they are holding back to assess the situation, the 'real person' is not allowed to emerge yet. They are testing the water to work out their role in the group and what behaviour is or is not acceptable.

The storming stage is when members begin to become more self-assured and possibly demanding. As a result they can become quite hostile towards each other as well as the therapist, asserting themselves and trying to find their place within the group.

During the norming stage the group has come to terms with itself and members have resolved some of the conflicts between them. Rules, both written and unwritten, are established as the group becomes more cohesive. A more intimate atmosphere develops, as group members get to know each other and the process becomes more trusting.

The performing stage can begin when the group has developed a collective identity. This is the time when serious work on the more sophisticated group tasks can begin. Its members are able to work easily and usefully together and group effectiveness is at its peak.

Therapists' behaviour should be matched to these stages. In order to help the group to make the best possible use of the time they have at their disposal, therapists should strive to develop a relaxed but task-oriented atmosphere within the group. This will help participants to develop norms and belief systems which are pertinent to the group goals and nurture constructive interaction between members. The therapist will need to gel the group in order for it to become a cohesive working unit. However, participants develop different positions within the group with respect to influence, being liked and disliked, and these differences can be used to good effect when developing communication within the group. It is important for therapists at all stages to be sensitive not only to communication content but to group process. The sensitivity towards the emotions of group members enables the therapist to give appropriate feedback, at later stages she might even confront members with certain aspects of their behaviour of which they are not aware.

Structure is a necessary part of group interaction. During the first phases of the group it is probably most helpful to start with more structure, but during later stages it will be more profitable to hand some of the leadership over to group members, which will increase their problem solving abilities.

In order to achieve the group's overall goals, interventions should be arranged according to a planned curriculum that outlines the sequences of behaviours expected of group members as they progress from the first through to the final session. Homework tasks should be set at the end of a session and participants will be expected to record their successes and failures for discussion at the following session.

Each group member will have his own particular problems as far as interaction is concerned and will need the opportunity to try to overcome them. The last few sessions of a group should be devoted to this purpose with each individual identifying the specific difficulties that are still causing him concern. These situations are then broken down for behavioural rehearsal where the other group members will be of assistance. Using group members in this way gives them also the opportunity of trying out different social interaction styles.

Therapists, as well as participants, often have difficulty preparing for the end of the group and this should be dealt with carefully when planning the group. The life cycle of the group should be clear to everyone from the beginning in order to control dependency on the group.

In order to lower reliance on the therapy procedure, the therapist will need to facilitate the client's ability to develop his own coping strategy. 'Rescuing' clients from difficult situations is the responsibility of the group leader only in the early stages, if at all. Ultimately it is in the client's best interests to use the difficulties as learning experiences which help to identify 'weaknesses' that could be targeted throughout the group.

Practical Suggestions for Leading the Group

The size of a group depends on the caseload, the needs of the clients and the goals in therapy. A group can be as small as two or three people or as large as eight. It seems more beneficial that members of groups should have a similar speech and language disorder, e.g. a stammering group, a dysphasia group, or a voice group, as clients with similar needs might be a better source of mutual support, mutual aid and problem solving.

Depending on the goals, therapists have to consider other variables concerning group composition such as age, gender and cultural background. It may be difficult to maintain an appropriate balance between homogeneity and heterogeneity. Group leaders will need to rely on their own clinical experience when making these decisions. Ideally, the membership of a social skills group would remain closed, i.e. stable during the life of the group. However, in certain situations, e.g. in a classroom setting, this might not be practical and the group would have to operate in a more flexible manner. It is important that the group members' expectations are commensurate with the aims of the group. Potential members will need basic information on the methods that are to be used and what is expected of them, e.g. active participation in the exercises; group rules have to be explained and agreed, e.g. that all information divulged in the group is confidential.

Running a group with a co-worker who could be from the same or an allied profession is the most helpful model. The group leaders will need to agree about how they will organize and run the group. They also need to understand each other's strengths and weaknesses and develop a high level of trust between them before they can instigate such feelings from their group members. It would therefore be important for them to spend some time together prior to embarking on any group interaction. The leaders should prepare the room prior to the group session so that there are the correct number of seats (one for each group member) arranged in a complete circle. Retaining the group circle is necessary, particularly following the 'breaking' of the group for an exercise.

Group gelling is of prime importance and breakdown within groups is often caused because not enough time has been spent on this task. The start of each session should contain group gelling exercises which can be achieved either through some of the exercises described in Chapter 9 or some other sharing opportunity, such as splitting the group into pairs or triads to discuss their homework tasks or when one person from each small group reports back to the leader and the rest of the group.

It is necessary for the group leader to ensure that all members of the group participate, and care will need to be taken of the more withdrawn members. Because of the importance of communication in the group, all activities will need to be encouraged whereby group members assist each other in attaining their individual goals. This can be achieved through small group work or 'pairing'.

Group members can work with a partner who will assist them in the group. This could be two reticent members working together to become more assertive within the group, or one more verbal member being asked to help a less able partner.

Important aspects of group leadership include the following:

1. Be prepared for the meeting (ensure materials, etc. are organized).
2. Ensure information is provided and information from the group is obtained.
3. The group leader should speak clearly, at the right time, and what is said should be related to what went on before; group members' interest must be held.
4. All members must be encouraged to participate (interaction should be primarily among members, and not dominated by the group leader or by particular group members).
5. The group leader should keep the interaction goal-directed and concrete.
6. The group leader should show warmth, genuineness and empathy.
7. The group leader should identify problems and deal with them.
8. Limits must be set when necessary.
9. The group leader should demonstrate, and give examples of strategies or interventions.
10. The group leader should praise effectively, note positive achievements of group members, and facilitate mutual praise among members.

A therapist's skill in the management of individual cases is useful in group therapy but the therapist should avoid treating group members individually within the group setting, i.e. making other group members act as observers as they wait their own turn. Thus, a therapist needs to be flexible and able to adapt to changes within the group and understand the strategies required to maintain the group's interest and cohesion.

A high level of concentration from group leaders is essential — they need to be sensitive, both to the individual group member's needs as well as those of the group as a whole. Good observational skills, the ability to view the group objectively, honesty and a sense of humour are skills that the therapist will find invaluable.

Goldstein *et al.* (1980) differentiate between general and specific trainer skills. General skills are those that are needed for success in practically every training, teaching or therapeutic effort:

- Oral communication and teaching ability.
- Flexibility and resourcefulness.
- Enthusiasm.
- Ability to work under pressure.
- Interpersonal sensitivity.
- Listening skills.
- Knowledge of human behaviour, adolescent development.

Specific trainer skills relate to the ability to set up structured experience in the behaviourist fashion:

- Knowledge of cognitive behavioural therapy, background, procedures, goals.
- Ability to train co-therapists.
- Ability to plan and present live modelling displays.
- Ability to initiate and sustain role playing.
- Ability to present material in concrete, behavioural form.
- Ability to deal with behavioural problems effectively.
- Accuracy and sensitivity in providing correct feedback.

It is also important that therapists are fully committed to their group in order to help group members become equally involved. Without firm commitment, therapy and social skills, training will not be successful. Flexibility and creativity enhance any changes that need to occur during an activity. The strength to confront problems and the courage to take some risks when appropriate makes the group lively and improves group dynamics.

In order to feel comfortable working in groups, leaders should have some strategies regarding their own problem solving techniques when difficulties arise. Below are some common problems encountered in groups and some suggestions for management.

A Group Member is Often Late

Being late can indicate many things. In the main it is lack of commitment to the group and needs to be taken seriously. If group leaders allow members to arrive whenever they please, then they must have a rationale for this 'rule' and to be comfortable that people entering and leaving the group at their will are not disrupting the rest of the group. If the rule of the group is that it will start promptly at 9.30 a.m. and this is agreed by the members including the leaders, then a late-comer must be dealt with:

- Take him on one side at the end of the session. Remind him of the rules of the group regarding time-keeping and listen carefully to his explanation. If a serious mishap has occurred, then this would have to be taken into account. If not, the group leader could ask him how he should deal with the problem of managing his erratic time-keeping.
- Take the problem to the group and let them resolve it.
- Suggest that the present group is not able to deal with this constant disruption and exclude the late-comer from further participation. This will require the leaders to 'repair' the broken group through discussion.

A Group Member Does Not Wish to Participate

- Take the problem to the group.
- Suggest that one member of the group 'looks after' the non-participator for a selected period of time.
- Take the client on his own to discuss his particular difficulty of working in the group.
- Ask him to sit next to a group leader for some of the time so that he feels he will not be 'left out'.

One Member Constantly Interrupts Group Dynamics

If one member of the group persistently interrupts the group proceedings, it can seriously affect the dynamics of the group, and the group leaders will need to address themselves to this difficulty. In the first instance, the leaders would need to hypothesize as to why the member was behaving in this way:

- Is the client highly anxious?
- Does the client understand the workings of the group?
- Is it a distracting device which can be a form of sabotage?

Action could include the following:

- Discuss the problem with the individual on his own.
- Do several turn-taking exercises and then discuss with the group.
- Encourage other members to be more active and avoid eye gaze with the disruptor.
- It is sometimes necessary to tell him to let others have their say.

A Group Member Chats to a Neighbour and does not Concentrate on Group Interaction

- If conversation is related to the group topic and the member is too shy to report in front of the large group then the leaders should encourage him to share his comments with the group.
- If the conversation has no relevance to the topic being discussed within the group, then leaders will need to stop this distracting behaviour:

  - discuss the problem within the group,
  - speak to the couple on their own and inform them that their individual chatting is sabotaging their own and other group members' therapy session,
  - with children, a 'time-out' system can be put into operation, i.e. exclude the offending distractor for one minute from the group activity.

Conflict within the Group

Squabbles can break out between group members and this needs to be dealt with openly and sensitively — confront problems rather than ignore them. Sometimes when group members feel successful at taking responsibility for themselves they may challenge the therapist's control and leadership position. Instead of quietly accepting more and more responsibility, members often feel the need to assert their new feelings of independence through rebellion and this can be regarded as a healthy and positive state.

It is important that leaders are aware of any members of a group who have reading and writing difficulties, if tasks requiring these skills are being set. Issues regarding smoking and swearing should be discussed with group members when setting down the 'rules' of the group.

It is helpful when running children's and adolescents' groups that disruptive behaviour is clearly defined so that members fully understand what is unacceptable.

Following an exercise, the group should reform their circle and time should be allowed for discussion of feelings, attitudes and outcome.

When dealing with clients' problems, the leaders will need to listen carefully to them and should communicate their willingness to help. Focus should be on the present crisis, and language should be direct and at the client's level. The problem should be sorted out into manageable parts and help given to decide what needs to be done. Alternative action and the consequences should be weighed up carefully and choices should be attainable as well as limited. Clients should be encouraged to do things for themselves as positive action, however small, brings about better feelings.

Example of a Group Programme

Social skills programmes can be run in conjunction with speech and language therapy intervention or as an entity in their own right as part of a package of care. It is possible for therapists to organize a programme to the specific needs of their clients as appropriate. The following guidelines can be easily adapted to most client groups and consist of eight sessions of approximately 90 minutes each. All the exercises can be found in Chapter 9.

Session 1

- The therapist supplies name tags for each person, if necessary, and presents an outline of the course and information regarding how the sessions will be managed regarding timing, cohesion, goals and homework tasks, etc.
- Perform exercise 11 — Finding out. This is a gelling exercise which will 'break the ice' for the participants. It is also the start of each person talking in the group and this is made easier for group members because they introduce their partner to the group rather than themselves.
- If the clients are to be assessed then this will need to be carried out during the first session (see Chapter 8).
- What are the expectations of the clients and therapist? Check if these are realistic and compatible. Break the group into pairs, or units of approximately four to five to discuss their expectations. These should then be shared with the whole group, giving the therapist the opportunity to ensure the expectations are realistic. The therapist can then discuss his own expectations of the group regarding, for example, time keeping, completing homework tasks, confidentiality regarding fellow members, etc.
- A discussion should follow regarding the goals of the programme and the importance of completing the homework tasks, which will be set at the end of each session and reviewed at the beginning of the next session.
- Perform exercise 54 — The name game. This is a second gelling exercise and helps members of the group to remember each other's names.
- Perform exercise 70 — Observations. This exercise enables group members to try out their observational skills in an unthreatening way and should be followed by a short group discussion as to how they felt and the purpose of the exercise.
- Brainstorm — why do we need observation in communication? How can we improve our observation skills?
- Record a short video of group members interacting in twos or threes and play it back. Participants should observe one good thing they are doing, and then something they need to change.

- Set homework: (1) to perform an observation exercise on four to six separate occasions with someone in their home or school, and (2) to observe and make notes of how people communicate — what is good or less desirable.
- End with feedback from all members of the group of how each individual felt about the session.

Session 2

- Review homework. Ensure it has been carried out and, if not, what have been the problems.
- Perform gelling exercise 25 — Introductions. This warm-up exercise will give group members the opportunity to hear everyone's name again.
- Relaxation should be introduced and the method of relaxation should be appropriate for the client group (see page 50). Discuss how relaxation is helpful in communication and how group members can transfer this into some situations outside the group.
- Perform exercise 1 — The listening exercise. This exercise should be carried out three times so that each member of a triad has a turn at telling an incident, listening and reporting back the incident, and making a judgement about the listener. A discussion should follow and each member can inform the group what they learned for themselves during the exercise. For example, a group member reported that he found the exercise difficult because he could remember the first part but forgot the final part of the incident that he was to listen to.
- Brainstorm — why is listening important in communication? What skills do we require to be good listeners? How can we improve our ability to listen.
- Perform turn-taking exercise 15 — Let me in. This exercise should be carried out only once within the triad. It gives the group members insight into how communication breaks down when people do not observe turn-taking rules. Each group member should describe how he felt in the role he was assigned (mother, father or child).
- Brainstorm — The role of turn-taking in communication and how it can be improved.
- Video session — Divide the group into sets of three. Each group is instructed to negotiate for something prescribed by the therapist according to age and ability. The videos are then viewed by the whole group and each member should report one positive thing he has seen and one skill he needs to improve.
- Set homework (for example): (1) to perform listening exercise three or four times during the week with family or friends, and (2) to concentrate on better turn-taking for 5 minutes, four times during the week.
- Group feedback.

Session 3

- Review homework, discuss any problems regarding listening and turn-taking.
- Perform gelling exercise 24 — Greetings.
- Perform relaxation exercise.
- Perform first praise exercise 29 — The praise game.
- Perform second praise exercise 67 — The praise circle.
- Brainstorm — The importance of praise and reinforcement in communication. Give full instructions on how to give and receive praise (this will be different for adults and children).
- Set homework (for example): (1) to praise a member of the family daily, (2) to perform relaxation (four to six times) — make a tape for each member if required, (3) to spend 5 minutes, four to six times during the week, concentrating on observation, listening and turn-taking, and (4) to think of a problem he has for the next session.

Session 4

- Review homework. Write down all problems.
- Perform exercises for confidence building, exercises 72, 65 and 56. Confidence is an important part of successful communication and these exercises allow group members to help each other to improve their self-esteem.
- Problem solving — choose one of the problems presented and carry out exercises.
- Set homework: (1) to perform relaxation, (2) to carry out problem solving exercise in home setting, (3) to praise a member of the family daily and note their response, and (4) to practise for 5 minutes four or five times during the week concentrating on observation, listening and turn-taking.
- Group feedback.

Session 5

- Review homework.
- Perform exercise 44 — Remember the objects. This exercise brings together gelling, memory, observation, turn-taking and co-operation.
- Discuss negotiation, brainstorm what is required, distribute hand-outs (p. 106).
- Make second negotiation video — small groups of two to three to work out a meal that they could make for a special occasion.
- Observe videos — each participant to make one positive statement and to decide on something else they would like to improve.
- Perform exercise 52 — I'm going to a party; for problem solving individually. This exercise requires each member to work out the rule of

the exercise without any assistance from other group members.
- Set homework: (1) to perform relaxation, (2) to problem solve in home setting, and (3) to concentrate for 5 minutes (four to six times) on changes they have decided to make after viewing negotiation video.
- Group feedback.

Negotiation – A Model

Negotiation is : a process for dealing with differences.
: a compromise.
Negotiation is NOT: an attack or battle which is won.

(1) Prepare
Don't jump straight in. Sit back and consider the following:

'What do I want to achieve?'
'What is the *least* I will be satisfied with?'
'What is the *most* I would like to gain?'

Consider how you would answer these questions *and* how the other person would answer them. Separate the people from the problem, and face the problem. Brainstorm.

(2) Discuss
Both sides put across their viewpoints and positions. *Listen* to the other person's side. Look out for signals that some compromise could be achieved. Do not simply argue over positions.

(3) Bargain
Begin to make suggestions of compromise.

'Perhaps if . . . . then maybe . . . .'

Look for mutual gain. Reason, and be open to reason.

(4) Decide
Make concrete agreements. Try to offer something which is valuable to the other person, but not too valuable for you to lose. Be prepared to make some concessions.

'if . . . . . . then . . . . . .'

Session 6

- Review homework tasks.
- Perform exercise 18 — Mode of transport. This exercise aims to help participants identify their moods and to verbalize them in a less

threatening way. It helps them to understand their own feelings as well as those of other group members.

- Discussion on how behaviour can change according to one's emotional state and how to be more perceptive regarding the feelings of others.
- Perform exercise 26 — Who feels the same? This exercise gives members the opportunity to practise various emotional states.
- Relaxation session followed by discussion of any problems that individuals might be experiencing.
- Discussion and preparation for disbanding the group after next session. Participants should divide into groups of two to four according to the number within the main group and be given time to discuss their feelings about the intended ending of the sessions. They should then formulate plans to support each other for the period from the end of the course to the follow-up day. For example, agree to telephone a group member enquiring how things are going for him, arrange to meet each other for tea or coffee, perhaps organize an outing for the whole group, etc. All participants then re-form to circle and share their experiences.
- Group to decide on video practice to be carried out. During these videos the therapist should help individual members with any difficulties through shaping and modelling as appropriate.
- Video feedback with individual advice to each group member, which he should record.
- Set homework: (1) to perform relaxation, (2) to give individual talks from video feed-back, (3) to increase the time (four to six times per week) when they put into practice all the social skills elements they have covered on the course, and (4) to bring any interaction problems they are experiencing for discussion at the next and last sessions.
- Group feedback. *See* Negotiation – A Model p.67.

Session 7

- Review homework.
- Note problems that have been reported and need to be worked on during the session.
- Perform exercise 87 — Do I look good? This exercise will help members to make positive statements as well as negative ones to others. A discussion should follow on how to deal with criticism.
- Set up a series of role plays using interaction problems reported during homework review.
- Preparation for homework tasks and group support system to be carried out until the follow-up session, which should take place in six to eight weeks.
- Social goodbye coffee 'party'.

- Homework tasks: (1) to set individual goals for each group member, (2) to perform relaxation, (3) to carry out agreed support to other group members, and (4) to spend short periods daily concentrating on skills learned during the course. Participants to send therapist a weekly report on their progress. Therapist to respond appropriately in writing.

Session 8 — Follow up

- Review homework tasks.
- Divide group into pairs to discuss with each other how they managed during the break, concentrating on the positive aspects rather than the negative.
- Couples to report back to the whole group. Therapist reinforcing and encouraging participants as appropriate and making a note of any serious problems which group members may have encountered.
- Divide group into two to discuss what they would like from this follow-up session and how they can maintain their newly acquired interaction skills. Follow by full group discussion.
- Carry out requests from group as appropriate.
- Role play solutions from reported difficulties.
- Set homework tasks on an individual basis: (1) to carry out support to other group members as agreed, and (2) to send report in writing to therapist in four weeks' time and he will respond appropriately.

Self-Help Groups

What are the options for long-term support after the therapy group has ended? Shortage of staff and financial pressures do not always permit therapists to give group members as much follow-up as would be desirable. Therefore therapists should consider referring at least some of the group members to a self-help group, or even initiate one themselves. It could be a profitable means of generalizing newly acquired skills as well as enabling clients to continue to work on problems which have been covered during the group.

The bedrock of self-help groups is that all its members share a common problem or concern. This common experience is crucial in helping members feel less isolated and to let them know they are not alone. What makes these groups unique is that the supporter and supported, or helper and helped are 'in the same boat', they are people who understand each other's problem. From this foundation, self-help groups develop their specific role in the fields of prevention or coping with chronic conditions. Self-help can and should be complementary to professional services, not a reaction against or an alternative to them.

If there are no self-help groups available in the area for a specific speech and language disorder, therapists might consider setting up a group. Members should eventually take over the control and running of the groups themselves (if appropriate) as quickly as possible in order to avoid an unhealthy dependency on the therapist.

An ongoing sensitive relationship between a professional and a group can be of great benefit, as therapists can give help and/or advice occasionally. Volunteers or aides can also be of value in helping to run and maintain self-help groups, particularly for neurologically impaired patients.

During the first phase of group development therapists might decide to be more than just supportive. Increasingly, it is being recognized that skills of leadership are necessary for self-help groups. Therapists might assist with helping the group to develop its goals and to share out the tasks and functions which can be undertaken by the members. Finding participants who are prepared to shoulder some of the responsibility is very important, as many groups experience difficulties, mainly with apathy. A great deal of effort can be expended on a group which ulti- mately fails because people are happy to let others 'get on with it'. Another threat to group cohesion which needs to be addressed is a possible lack of mutual tolerance. The group has to give itself specific norms in order to survive. On the other hand, group members should respect each other and avoid ostracism. Of course, care should be taken that self-help groups are not too cosy, which might inhibit change. These dangers should be pointed out to groups at the outset and group members should discuss and find ways to avoid these problems. Some groups might choose not to have a leader but to share the responsibil- ities between them. Others might decide to have a different leader at each meeting thus giving everyone a chance to develop leadership skills. It is now well recognized that the skills of leadership are necessary for self-help groups to be successful and perhaps the therapist should be involved in such training.

Chapter 6
Social Skills Training for the Speech and Language Impaired

Introduction

Speech and language impaired people are under more stress than the normal population. Constant pressure can cause the development of undesirable forms of behaviour that go beyond the limitation of the speech and language impairment. Emotional tension can arise when the environment fails to meet the needs of the individual or when events or situations are construed as 'threatening'. Furnham (1986) noted that non-handicapped people tend to interact relatively infrequently with handicapped individuals because of their negative attitudes. They perceive the handicapped individual as dependent, isolated, depressed, emotionally unstable and socially inadequate (Furnham and Pendred, 1983).

Handicapped people are often denied the opportunity to observe and practise 'normal' social skills interaction. In order to address this problem, social skills training programmes have been developed for handicapped people to:

> increase their rates of positive social interaction, decrease rates of negative social interaction, and/or enhance their social accept-ance by non-handicapped peers (Gresham, 1981).

It would seem, therefore, that the training of social skills for handi-capped people would be helpful in enabling them to be more adept in interacting with their peers as well as the normal population. This would include speech and language impaired people who are often unable successfully to initiate and maintain interactions.

Many children with a speech/language impairment have inadequate social skills. Poor attention control may lead to impaired listening and turn-taking skills, and memory. Problems with initiation, topic mainten-ance and termination may arise from inadequate linguistic skills as well as social withdrawal and passivity. In developing a social skills training

71

programme for children, it is essential to involve and train the parents as they provide a model, give emotional support and play a crucial role in interpreting life events for their children. Moore (1967) views parental involvement as a key factor for a child to be well adjusted. Only if parents have mastered various skills are they able to act as a model and teach their children, thereby reinforcing skills taught to the child in the clinical setting.

Specific Language Impairment

Specific language impairment is a term used to describe the language profile of a particular group of children. Goldstein and Gallagher (1992, p. 8 – 9) describe it as follows: 'Specific language impairment (SLI) is a developmental language disability that is not attributable to any of the major disabling conditions that account for other types of language disability. Children with SLI do not have clinically significant sensory, intellectual, neurological, emotional or oral–motor impairments . . .'. However, despite considerable research, it has not been possible to identify a common aetiology for these children and therefore SLI continues to be defined by exclusion criteria as indicated above rather than by positive indicators. Within this heterogeneous group there is a subgroup of children who have particular difficulty in understanding and using the rules of social interaction. These children have been described as having pragmatic or, in some cases, semantic–pragmatic difficulties. Adams and Bishop (1989) and Bishop and Adams (1989) provide a useful summary of the language characteristics of these children as outlined below:

Pragmatic Problems I: Violation of exchange structure. This category includes children who have difficulty with taking conversational turns. They may either not respond at all or ignore the other person's contribution and continue talking on an unrelated topic.

Pragmatic Problems II: Failure to use context in comprehension. These children experience difficulty interpreting abstract or more idiomatic language appropriately. The child responds to the literal meaning of the utterance and fails to understand its implied meaning, e.g. teacher: "Do you want to go out at playtime?" (said in response to inappropriate behaviour, i.e. a threatened sanction), child: "Yes" (and continues to behave in the same way).

Pragmatic Difficulties III: Too little information given to partner. The child misjudges how much the listener knows about the topic and assumes that they know far more than they do, e.g. child: "He said to her not to go there" (the listener has no information about the people or the place).

Pragmatic Problems IV: Too much information provided to partner. The child is unable to modify his utterances in relation to previous discussions/shared knowledge. The child overelaborates in response to simple questions and has difficulty bringing the conversational turn to an end.

Clearly, this behaviour is not atypical of many young children. However, children with persistent difficulties in this area can be identified by the extent to which their language has these characteristics and the perseverance of this trait beyond the age when other children have begun to modify their conversational skills.

Voice Disorders

The voice is just one component of communicative competence; however, a deficit of one skill often affects or is affected by deficits in other areas. Vocal competence is determined by the way the individual adapts vocal behaviour to individual needs, the reaction of others, and the constraints of their communicative environment. Interpersonal factors that can influence vocal behaviour may include when and how much to talk, when not to talk, the volume and pitch that are appropriate, and the use of the voice in expressing emotion. A breakdown in these skills may either contribute to the development of a dysphonia or to its maintenance. Other important social skills that enhance effective vocal behaviour are awareness of feedback from others (e.g. eye-contact, listening skills), sharing talking time, and awareness of other people's needs.

It is therefore important for clinicians to evaluate the role interpersonal factors play in dysphonic patients' vocal strategies and their effects on their interaction with others.

Laryngectomy patients often have great difficulty coming to terms with change in their method of communication and their altered physical appearance. Close friends and relatives are frequently distressed by these changes, which they have to learn to accept in order for new methods of communication to be explored. Therapists report that laryngectomy patients can become more demanding while engaging in conversation which disrupts turn-taking. They often develop poor eye gaze which enables them to continue talking by not picking up non-verbal cues from the listener to relinquish their turn.

Although many patients with voice disorders exhibit inappropriate social skills there is little evidence of the use of social skills training with this group. Furthermore, there is little research available regarding the extent to which poor social skills affect the development or maintenance of a voice disorder. Despite this paucity of evidence, we feel that considering and treating social skills deficits as an integral part of a voice disorder is a clinically valid target of intervention.

Deafness

Deafness itself does not imply any consequent social impairment. In support of this Groce (1985) describes the unusual social history of Martha's Vineyard from the 17th century to the early years of the 20th century, when there was an extremely high incidence of profound hereditary deafness. As a result, sign language was widely used in the hearing as well as the deaf community. This resulted in complete and successful integration of deaf people into the social life of the island. More commonly, however, deaf people formed and still form small minority groups. At present the incidence of severe deafness at birth is approximately 1 in 1000, and 90 – 95% of deaf children are born into hearing families. The difficulties that deaf people experience with social skills arise from having to integrate with the hearing, speaking majority.

Deaf people have difficulties in accessing and acquiring spoken language. Even children with mild to moderate losses can have significantly delayed spoken language (Davis, 1986). Many social interactions are dependent on linguistic ability (McTear, 1991) and so deaf children often have difficulties with spoken interactions because of immature vocabulary and syntax. For example, they may have a limited vocabulary of words used to greet people and initiate conversations. Therefore speech and language therapists often combine social skills training with therapy involving other aspects of language such as vocabulary building.

Interactions between deaf children and hearing people are often controlled by the hearing partner. For example, Wood et al. (1982) found that teachers of deaf children exhibited high levels of control which negatively correlated with the length of children's contributions and degree of initiative. This control is often used to avoid conversational breakdown but it does not allow deaf children to take responsibility for their own communicative effectiveness, and limits their ability to develop effective social skills with hearing people. Deaf people are often required to engage in difficult social situations with hearing people and may not be prepared for or have the sophisticated skills necessary for dealing with them satisfactorily. Beazley (1992) gives examples of how social skills training can help deaf people to reflect constructively on previous unsuccessful interactions with hearing people and prepare for future interactions. She discusses the important role that group social skills training has in providing these experiences and describes a programme based on the categories described in this book, i.e. foundation, interactive, affective and cognitive skills.

Mental Illness

Social skills training has been for many years an integral part of rehabilitation programmes for clients with mental health problems (e.g.

Marzillier and Winter, 1978). However, a growing number of speech and language therapists are now increasingly involved with this client group. This development has led to more collaboration within multidisciplinary teams and has led to wider recognition of the expertise that the speech therapist can bring to acute and rehabilitative settings in the community. The provision of therapy programmes for clients, and needs-based training for support staff, has opened up areas for research into many aspects of the development of social language and its deterioration during mental illness.

Mental illness can affect communication in a wide variety of ways. In addition, drug-induced involuntary movement disorders, such as tardive dyskinesia, frequently lead to increased social difficulties outside the institutional context. It is also acknowledged that disturbances of speech and language can be indicative of deteriorating mental states.

Assessment procedures for the mentally ill focus particularly on attention and memory, perceptual and associative deficits, receptive and expressive language, as well as the pragmatic aspects of social communication. These contribute to an holistic view of the client's functional communication skills.

Therapy programmes generally involve regular group sessions which provide a safe setting in which participants may change their view of themselves as communicators, developing more flexible and effective ways of interacting as they receive validation and feedback from others (Hayes, 1997). They are offered opportunities to practise the skills of social interaction by taking part in facilitated communication activities, using techniques such as modelling/shaping, role play and video recording. Group members are involved in evaluating their own development, and supported in generalizing their skills into other settings. Individual therapy programmes cover a wide range of difficulties, including voice, fluency and articulation problems, as well as inappropriate social behaviour.

Acquired Neurological Disorders

Although there has been little research into the consequences of stroke or head injury with regard to social skills, it is generally accepted that all patients with acquired neurological disorders show some impairment of social skills function. The degree of disintegration of social skills will vary from one patient to another and factors such as social states, premorbid employment and social skills inability, as well as environment, will all affect the therapist's interpretation and assessment of the patient post trauma. In addition, the expectation and perceptions of the family and friends will need to be considered as they will be heavily involved in assisting the neurologically impaired patient in their rehabilitation.

When deciding on the social skills input into the speech and language therapy programme for this group of patients, an estimate will need to be made regarding the patient's potential prognosis and future lifestyle. If the patient is likely to return to work, whether in his premorbid capacity or at some other level, his social skills training needs will be different from the patient who is likely to remain at home or in long-term care.

Head Injury

Characteristically, head injury results in a severe disturbance of social skills. The degree to which social interaction is impaired will depend to some extent on the severity of the head injury and the site of the lesion. Many head-injured patients are disinhibited, have uncontrolled mood swings and are emotionally volatile. They are likely to have problems with all aspects of social skills and a comprehensive and intensive social skills training programme should be an integral part of the patient's rehabilitation.

Aphasia

Aphasic patients' verbal communication is disrupted and their comprehension of language as well as its expression may be affected. This has implications with regard to their ability with cognitive skills such as negotiation, assertion, problem solving, self-monitoring, evaluation and reinforcement. Interaction skills will also be severely affected. The patient's physical disability, possible facial palsy and decreased mobility can affect facial expression, posture and eye contact. This may lead to embarrassment in the patient and in the other people participating in the social interaction.

Patients have the added burden of becoming depressed following a stroke and this can also affect their presentation of themselves. Relatives and friends may misinterpret this as a general lack of interest, so they will need to be incorporated into the social skills training as well as the speech and language input.

Dysarthria

Patients presenting with dysarthria as a result of cerebral trauma, stroke or degenerative disease are likely to have problems of mobility and altered facial expression resulting from damage to the seventh cranial nerve. With regard to communication, this has implications for posture, facial expression and eye-contact.

Emotional lability is a common problem for patients with bulbar palsy and pseudo bulbar palsy. Such lability upsets the social interaction between the patient and others and frequently causes distress.

The slurred and sometimes unintelligible speech of dysarthrics can make them withdraw from social interaction and their altered voice prosody and intonation may be interpreted as a flattening of mood rather than being accepted as a characteristic of the speech impairment. Self-monitoring is a skill which will need to be developed by the patient.

Dysphagia

People with dysphagia may become socially withdrawn if they are too embarrassed to eat and drink with other people because of their swallowing difficulties. They may feel that they are 'messy' eaters with all the connotations attached to this. They will therefore need advice on improving mechanical skills, such as exercises to strengthen lip closure and to improve chewing (if this is appropriate). It may be helpful for the person to discuss their embarrassment openly with family and friends.

If the person is deemed completely unsafe for eating and drinking then this obviously also precludes any opportunity for social interaction in this context. If the person is in hospital the relatives will be unable to show their care and concern for the patient by bringing in things for them to eat. Both of these aspects may increase the person's isolation and it is therefore useful to liaise with ward staff, relatives and other team members to discuss ways of preventing this.

Learning Disability

There is a high level of social skills deficit within the learning disabled population (Hitchings and Spence, 1991). Therefore social communication skills training is a key area to be incorporated into the speech and language therapy programme. This group experiences the same delay in social skills development as they do in all other areas of their learning but they respond well to a comprehensive social skills training programme (Matson et al., 1980).

It is essential that any social skills training should be tailored to the abilities of the learning disabled person, and Hitchings and Spence (1991) include an assessment procedure that measures clients' non-verbal and verbal skills.

The speech and language therapist is involved with this client group from pre-school to adulthood, and is responsible for designing training programmes to meet individual needs (Rinaldi, 1992). Therapists are also involved in training parents and siblings to be good models of social interaction in the home environment as this plays an important role in supporting the skills that the children are learning in therapy. Once in school or an adult training centre, teachers, carers and staff need to be involved in training that will enable them to support and encourage the use of social communication skills within these environments (Kelly, 1996).

Stuttering

Current literature on social skills training makes little reference to the problem of stuttering. However, it is widely acknowledged that many stutterers demonstrate deficits in social skills. These do not appear at the time of onset, which is usually between the ages of $2^1/_2$ and 6 years, but may become increasingly evident as the normal process of social communication is disrupted by the breakdown in fluency. There is a growing body of evidence, both clinical and research based, that the nature of the interaction between a stuttering child and his family plays an important role in the development and maintenance of the problem. Teaching parents to re-evaluate and make small changes in their social interaction skills has proved a powerful tool in the early remediation of stuttering (Rustin *et al.*, 1996). There are many factors that have been shown to be influential and these include observation and listening skills, rate of speech, directiveness, and reducing the complexity of inter-actions. For older children, where the stuttering has become more firmly established, it begins to affect their ability to deal with a wide range of social situations. Repeated experience of communicative breakdown results in stutterers having increasing difficulties with social adjustment (Bloodstein, 1995). Rustin (1984) demonstrated the contribution that social skills training can make in the treatment of adolescent stutterers on a two-week intensive course. This study compared the outcome of three treatment groups in terms of improvement and maintenance of fluency as well as reduction in perceived stress levels and increased confidence. The therapy programme for one group consisted of fluency technique training only, the therapy programme for a second group was social skills training only, and a third group were given a combined programme of technique and social skills training. The results at one-year follow-up showed that the combined group were the most fluent and showed the least anxiety. Whilst there was some difference between the fluency of the technique group and the social skills group, there was less perceived anxiety recorded in the social skills only group.

As a result of this research, programmes have been developed for 9 – 18 year-olds that include social skills as an important integral part of the treatment process (Rustin, 1987; Rustin *et al.*, 1995).

Chapter 7
Developing Social Communication Skills within the Mainstream School Context

By Claire Topping, *Principal Speech and Language Therapist for Mainstream Schools, Camden and Islington Community NHS Trust*

Introduction

In England and Wales, the Education Act of 1981 heralded a new approach towards children with significant special educational needs (SEN). Rather than using a diagnostic label to identify a child's educational placement, a profile of need was to be drawn up, based on a multidisciplinary assessment. From this information, the most suitable provision would be identified. In addition, the emphasis was towards educating children within mainstream school classes whenever possible. A statement identifying the child's special educational needs, and the provision that would be made available to meet them, was then issued. One of the prime reasons for placing children with SEN in mainstream schools is to give them opportunities to observe and interact with children who provide models of appropriate learning and social behaviours. To this end the underlying philosophy and management of the school is crucial to the development of appropriate social communication skills. Clear school guidelines around behaviour management and playground protocol can help to provide an environment where positive models can be demonstrated. In addition, the attitude of staff to each other will also provide models of behaviour for all children. As Ross and Ryan (1990) note in their work on improving primary school playgrounds, 'It is important that the children perceive non-teaching staff to be awarded the same respect as teachers in order to combat the notion that some people matter less than others and can be treated with less consideration . . . A staff which is seen to collaborate (as opposed to working completely in isolation) can offer a strong model of people working together for a common good . . .'.

Recent legislation (e.g. The Education Act of 1993 and the subsequent Code of Practice, 1994), has extended the earlier act (which had focused on the 2 per cent of children with most severe needs), to include all children who might present with special educational needs. It advocated a staged approach within which children could be supported by a range of means depending upon their level of need. The school is seen as central to the management of the child's needs, with a nominated person, the Special Educational Needs Co-ordinator (SENCo), responsible for ensuring that the school provides the appropriate support. Children at stage two and above of the Code of Practice, must have an individual education plan (IEP), which has specific targets, which are monitored and updated on a regular basis.

Increasing numbers of children with significant special educational needs now attend mainstream schools. This presents school staff with both opportunities and challenges in developing an environment from which these children can benefit both educationally and socially. Children with SEN highlight the need for good practice at every level of school organization, which in turn benefits all children at the school. In addition, many of the strategies developed by specialist/advisory staff to support these children dovetail with good teaching practice and link into issues that are relevant to the entire school population. For a class teacher in the larger classes of mainstream schools, it is important to identify the threads of commonality of need within the class as well as the specific needs of individual children. Social communication skills work provides a useful framework for identifying such commonality. Regardless of aetiology, many children require support in developing appropriate observation, listening, turn-taking, reinforcement and problem solving skills.

The National Curriculum was introduced following the Education Reform Act of 1988. Its aim is to provide a broad and balanced curriculum for all children regardless of placement within a mainstream or special school. In addition, the curriculum should offer a range of personal and social opportunities for each individual pupil so that he or she can contribute positively to society both as a child and as a future adult member of the community. Key areas of study were identified and different levels of attainment within each area identified. Social communication skills development links strongly with the speaking and listening targets within the National Curriculum.

For example:

- 'Participate as speakers and listeners in group activities . . .' Speaking and listening: Level one, attainment target (AT) 1.
- 'Give a detailed oral account of an event, or something that has been learnt in the classroom, or explain with reasons why a particular course of action has been taken.' Speaking and listening: Level four, AT1.
- 'Take part as speakers and listeners in group discussion or activity

expressing a personal view and commenting constructively on what is being discussed or experienced.' Speaking and listening: Level four, AT1.

- 'Contribute to and respond constructively in discussion, including the development of ideas, advocate and justify a point of view.' Speaking and listening: Level five, AT1.

In addition, personal and social education (PSE) explicitly mentions social development:

- '. . . the personal and social development of pupils is a major aim of education . . .'. NCC Guidance No. 3 (1990).

Fisher (1990) notes 'Today there is a greater emphasis on the *process* of learning, on investigation and *problem solving* (this author's italics), on reading for meaning, on use of *reasoning* in writing, on study skills and on developing autonomous ways of learning . . .'. This notion of 'process' or the means by which the curriculum content is learnt is a vital part of successful classroom management.

Developing Social Competence

Defining social competence is a complex task. The number of definitions is nearly equal to the number of researchers interested in the topic (Dodge, 1985). However, Guralnick (1992) notes that most definitions include elements of *effectiveness* in influencing a peer's social behaviour and *appropriateness* within a given context. Within the classroom, the socially ineffective child is often peripheral to the social system within the class, presenting as a rather passive and/or isolated member of the group. The child may attempt to engage with other children but does so in a manner that is either rejected by the peer group or makes it difficult to maintain the activity in question. With very young children the idea of 'entry' skills, i.e. the ability to initiate social interaction or break into an existing social dynamic had been explored by a number of researchers. Observation and imitation skills, perseverance and 'repair' skills (which can be considered to be early problem solving/negotiation skills) have been identified as factors affecting successful outcomes. There are six key factors that can be considered when facilitating communication skills within the classroom context.

1. The environment.

2. Adult/teacher communication style.

3. Individual child's communication style.

4. Child's compensation strategies for areas of difficulty.

5. The whole-class dynamic.

6. Opportunities for direct skill teaching within the context of small group work.

The Environment

When considering social communication skills development within the school/classroom context it is important to examine how different aspects of the environment can affect an individual child. The child may be experiencing difficulties in one, several or all aspects of the social structure within the school or classroom.

In primary school, children spend at least one-fifth of the school day in the playground, Ross and Ryan (1990). Observation of children during breaks can provide useful information about both individual children and the overall behaviour of children generally within this context. As always, it is important to consider the broader picture first. If playtime is generally an issue within the school, due to bullying or excessively rough games, the child with SEN will almost inevitably experience difficulties too. Investigating playground organization, Ross and Ryan (1990) state 'The problem of exclusion (from activities) relates to the boredom of the playground. If there are few activities and games on offer, children find it difficult to join in something else . . . Younger children, bilingual children and children with special educational needs all need to be considered when evaluating power relationships in the playground. Any individual child who is 'different' in some way . . . can be a target for bullying.' Playground organization can facilitate or impede the development of social competence. Structured activities such as skipping, 'grandmother's footsteps' or clapping games provide children with a framework of 'rules' and many such games develop skills of turn-taking, observing and listening. The provision of quiet areas where children can participate in small group activities away from the hurly burly of the more physical organized games such as football, will also facilitate interaction.

Within the classroom itself the layout, e.g. seating arrangements, and range of activities available, should also be considered. Odom et al. (1990) investigating early years classrooms, found that both children with and without disabilities engaged most in verbal social interaction during free play and tidying up activities. Stoneman et al. (1983) identified blocks/bricks, home corner and waterplay as promoting peer interaction.

For more formal discussion situations with older children, seating arrangements can facilitate the group's focus. An accurate circle of chairs enables all participants to see each other and bestows an immediate sense of equality for all group members. The absence of desks encourages a sense of openness. Depending on the purpose of the activity, the teacher may wish to be part of the circle, e.g. during whole class dynamic work, or act as a facilitator slightly outside the circle, e.g. encouraging peer–peer discussion. When one person is the major focus of an activity, e.g. whole class feedback by a spokesperson following small group discussion, the use of a semi-circle format around the speaker may be helpful.

Another aspect of the physical environment is noise level. At risk of stating the obvious, children and adults should be able to hear each other without the need to shout or ask for continual repetition. The provision of a quiet area within the room where discussion activities can take place will undoubtedly enhance the likelihood of a successful interaction, be it child to adult or peer to peer.

Adult/Teacher Communication Style

Vygotsky (1962) identified the zone of proximal development. This zone represents the difference between what the child can achieve unaided and what can be achieved with appropriate support from a peer or adult. The notion of verbal 'scaffolding' is derived from this theory. Scaffolding allows a child to achieve success in tasks he would not accomplish unaided. It acts as a prompt, encouraging the child to identify the next step to take. The level of scaffolding may vary depending on the needs of the child at a particular time. The examples below demonstrate different levels of modelling by the adult, with increasing responsibility gradually being transferred from the adult to the child:

- A six-year-old child who, although able to formulate short sentences, responds by screaming if a peer requests something such as borrowing a pencil.
- Adult scaffold (a): 'If you don't want him to have it say "No".'
- Adult scaffold (b): 'What do you say if you don't want him to have it?'
- Adult scaffold (c): 'Tell him if you don't want him to have it.'

The status of talk within the classroom and the communicative behaviour of individual teachers and other members of school staff will affect the social communication development of the child. Heatherington (1989), provides a teachers' self-evaluation checklist which asks a range of useful basic questions for self-evaluation. (See Table 7.1.)

Weitzman (1992) identifies six communication styles or 'roles' of adults/teachers when interacting with young children:

Table 7.1. Self evaluation Checklist for Teachers

Am I defeating good listening by talking too much?

Do I realize that children have difficulty listening attentively for a long period of time?

Do I vary my style of presentation in order to encourage children to listen?

Do I expect children to concentrate on too many things at once?

Do I give children the time to find the answer to one question before another one is asked?

Do I ask open-ended questions that do not require right or wrong answers?

Are my explanations clearly presented?

Do I try not to repeat what the child says, but rather require the class to concentrate on the child speaking?

Am I taking too much time in explaining to one child while others lose interest?

Do I try not to repeat phrases and expressions so often that they become ineffective and monotonous?

Do I treat children's opinions with respect?

Am I getting the full attention of the class before giving information?

Do I make myself available for listening?

Do children feel free to come to me with their problems and know that they will have my undivided attention?

Taken from: Heatherington, M., (1989) Listening and talking in year one. In J. Dwyer (Ed.), *A sea of talk* (pp 9 – 20). Rozelle: Primary English Teaching Association.

1. *The director role.* The adult maintains tight control over the children and the activities. Much time is spent in making suggestions, giving directions and asking questions. This makes it difficult for children to initiate and play an active role in interactions.
2. *The entertainer role.* The adult is playful and provides enjoyable activities but still does most of the talking and playing. Again, this provides little opportunity for the children to initiate and take an active part.
3. *The timekeeper role.* In this role the teacher rushes through activities and routines, allowing only very limited interactions to occur.
4. *The too-quiet role.* This time the child's attempts at initiating an interaction are not followed up.
5. *The rescuer–teacher role.* The teacher assumes that the child won't be able to express himself. The teacher speaks for the child or offers help before the child asks.

6. *The responsive teacher role*. The teacher is tuned into the individual child's interests and needs and responds in ways to encourage interaction with both peers and adults.

Weitzman (1992) has developed a training package called the Hanen programme which investigates how adults can develop their interactional styles to maximize communication development in young children.

In addition to conversational style considerations, each teacher has her own way of conveying information regarding expectations of the class group. This constitutes the 'hidden curriculum' of the classroom and includes a wide range of adult behaviours, e.g. how a teacher attracts attention, signals the end of an activity, responds to 'undesirable' behaviour, gives praise and uses humour. Many of these rules are never overtly stated and the majority of children can extract them from their own observations and are able to adapt as they move classes and change teachers. Children with SEN are much less likely to respond to these implicit communications and will benefit from much more structured and repeated explanation of class rules.

Individual Child's Style of Communication

Weitzman (1992) also identifies four communication styles for children. Although these styles were developed from working with very young children, they apply across a broad age range.

1. *The sociable child*. The child initiates interactions constantly and is very responsive to others' interactions.
2. *The reluctant child*. This child rarely initiates and is often on the outside of group activities and interactions. The child may take a long time to 'warm up' but will interact given sufficient time and opportunity.
3. *The child with his own agenda*. This child appears to lack interest in interaction. He may spend a lot of time playing independently and usually rejects efforts to engage him.
4. *The passive child*. The child seldom responds or initiates, and demonstrates little interest in the people or environment around him.

Child's Compensation Strategies for Areas of Difficulty

Increasingly, the 'medical' or 'deficit' model of communication difficulties is being superseded by one which, whilst still attempting to build specific skills, increasingly looks towards developing strategies that enable the child to compensate for what may, in some cases, be life-long difficulties. The emphasis is towards identifying the functional impact of an underlying disability and developing a programme of support to meet these functional needs. Strategies will vary depending on the precise nature of the child's difficulty but a key one is 'comprehension monitoring'. Comprehension monitoring can be described as children's ability actively to monitor their level of understanding by:

- Identifying *when* they have not understood.
- Identifying *why* they have not understood, e.g. talking too fast, sentence too long, unfamiliar vocabulary, etc.
- Providing *appropriate feedback* to the speaker, e.g. 'Please say it again', 'I don't know what "X" means', etc.

The development of such strategies may need to be addressed either prior to or alongside social communication skills work as described in this book. Commercially available programmes of comprehension monitoring are available for both primary and secondary aged children, e.g. Mancuso (1988) and Danielson and Sampson (1992).

The Whole-class Dynamic

An effective whole-class dynamic is fundamental to successful teaching and learning. If children are unable to work collaboratively to achieve a common goal, both the quality and quantity of their learning will be severely compromised. However, the need to provide structured opportunities so that children may learn the skills necessary for effective collaboration is sometimes overlooked within the teaching context. In trying to meet the needs of individual children, the needs and competence of the entire class group must be considered.

Curry and Bromfield (1994) provide practical guidance on developing the whole-class dynamic in primary schools via the use of circle-time. Circle-time has many parallels with the social communication skills approach and activities described in this book. Circle-time has been found to be particularly helpful in situations where the whole class is in need of support to develop socially appropriate and effective behaviour.

Stanford and Stoate (1990), when working with secondary-aged pupils, identified the following as characteristics of effective classsroom groups:

- The members understand and accept one another.
- Communication is open.

- Members take responsibility for their own learning and behaviour.
- Members co-operate.
- Processes for making decisions have been established.
- Members are able to confront problems openly and resolve their conflicts constructively.

In addition, five stages of group development within the classroom context are identified.

- Stage One: Orientation (gelling). The group members become acquainted and begin to understand why they are there.
- Stage Two: Establishing norms. These include norms for group responsibility, responsiveness to others, co-operation, decision making through consensus and confronting problems.
- Stage Three: Coping with conflict. The group learns how to deal constructively with conflict.
- Stage Four: Productivity. Group identity emerges and the group is at its most effective in achieving its aims and supporting the emotional needs of its members.
- Stage Five: Termination. The group ends and its members disperse.

Children will experience many group life-cycles during their school career and the incidence of these will rise rapidly upon transfer to secondary school, presenting a real challenge to both students and teachers in ensuring that effective group working is achieved in all subject areas.

Opportunities for Small Group Work

Research carried out in early years classrooms indicates that peer interaction is most likely to take place in small groups (two or three children) (Sainato and Carta, 1992). Adult led/facilitated structured small group work provides opportunities for a high level of practice for certain skills such as turn-taking. Children with limited attention control will benefit from the reduced waiting times between turns and are more likely to remain on task than in whole-class discussion activities. The use of small group work to support children with SEN is now well established within mainstream classes and provides an ideal forum to integrate the activities described in this book as part of children's individual education plan (IEP). Small group work can act as a 'bridge' towards whole class activities such as circle time. Complementary activities can be developed or, alternatively, the children can have opportunities to 'rehearse' to help them cue in more rapidly when the activities are presented to the whole group.

Summary

Social communication skill development forms an integral part of effective learning as well as developing appropriate social relationships with adults and children.

Whilst recognizing that individual children may experience particular difficulty with certain aspects of this skill, a child's ability to function successfully also depends on a number of other factors. Not least of these is the communicative behaviour of the adults and peers with whom he interacts on a regular basis.

Chapter 8
Theory and Practice in the Assessment of Social Skills

The goal of assessment is to measure social skills competence in order to define changes required in the client's social interaction. As social skills training has been derived from the behaviour therapy model, it would seem that a systematic and comprehensive analysis before and after treatment would give clinicians the necessary information about the effectiveness of their intervention procedures. However, assessment methodology in the field of social competence is unable to fully reflect the complexities of social interaction.

The parametric approach of behaviour therapy, e.g. measuring the length of eye-contact, is too simple for the multiple and complicated facets of human interaction. However, weakness in assessment instrumentation should not lead us to 'no assessment'. Only relatively objective measures will give us the opportunity to refine and develop our procedures further. Inappropriate assessment could lead to incorrect conclusions, resulting in suboptimal treatment.

Behavioural research on interpersonal behaviour has been based on the assumption that molar skill categories such as assertiveness are based on identifiable sets of molecular behaviours, e.g. voice volume and eye-contact. Even if this assumption has been generally supported in correlational studies, there is still little evidence, as a review of the literature shows, that the components typically assessed and subjected to treatment are important correlates of dysfunctional behaviour as it occurs in the natural environment. The question is not if the molecular responses like eye-contact or voice volume are relevant, but whether they are relevant in a specific situation. Therefore, assessment has to include the situational variable, i.e. the usual social context for the individual. The trainee has not only to know how to make certain responses but when and where.

There have been two basic ways of operationalizing competent social behaviours, either in terms of global evaluative criteria (molar) or as discrete, concrete and isolated responses which are part of a larger chain (molecular) behaviour. Although both models have been criticized, they do have their merits if they are not over-used. The molecular model is more precise but it makes predictions of behaviour in different settings difficult; the molar model allows cross-situational predictions but this gain in social validity has the drawback of lower reliability. It is important, therefore, that the behaviours which have been selected as 'target behaviours' are genuinely important in the subject's social environment. Socially invalid assessment might lead to training trivial behaviours. The social importance, the effectiveness and the functional utility of the selective behaviours need to be considered.

This theoretically complicated interactive model emphasizes the role of environmental variables, personal characteristics and their interactions, and is the only realistic approach to training.

Rinn and Markle (1979) categorized social skills into four repertoires which are a basic guideline to select the relevant variables for assessment:

1. *Self-expressive skills:* expression of feelings, e.g. sadness and happiness; expression of opinion; accepting compliments; making positive statements about oneself.
2. *Reinforcement skills:* making positive statements about a friend, stating genuine agreement with another's opinion, praising others.
3. *Assertive skills:* making simple requests, disagreeing with another's opinion, denying unreasonable requests.
4. *Communication skills:* conversing, interpersonal problem solving.

These skills may require simplification for specific groups of speech and language impaired patients; for instance, a severely mentally handicapped client with only the most rudimentary of social skills, or a stroke patient suffering from dyspraxia, word finding difficulties and uncontrollable drooling. Thus assessment and relevant treatment must take into account both the speech disorder and the behavioural problem. The significant features of each patient's specific abilities and disabilities will need to be identified and then incorporated into an individualized treatment programme.

The Practice of Assessment

The assessment of the client means different things to different clinicians, depending on their training and orientation. Psychodynamic therapists normally take a detailed life history with an emphasis on early development. Behaviour therapists concentrate on behaviour and cognition, focusing on current functioning.

The process of clinical decision-making has often been represented metaphorically as a funnel in which the scope of information gathered and the range of treatment options narrows as therapy progresses. The suitability of various treatment modalities and formats for altering the behaviour gets clearer as the specific nature of the presenting problem becomes apparent and is defined in concrete behavioural terms. This metaphor may capture some elements of the process but it is certainly an oversimplification, as it ignores not only the subtleties of the cognitive skills to select as a target for changing a specific behaviour, but also the common clinical fact that clients frequently reveal 'new' and important problems during the course of therapy. It would therefore appear to be more accurate to see the clinician's activities as a recursive, iterative problem solving and decision-making process. We have to be aware of the many factors that influence clinicians' decisions regarding how best to treat presenting problems: diagnosis, severity of problem, aetiologic considerations, consequences of selecting and altering target behaviours, competing problem behaviours, expected probability and degree of success, motivational and client resource issues, ethical considerations and possibilities for post-treatment maintenance of behavioural change.

Although there are commonalities among clients with speech disorders, no one programme fits every one of them. It is advisable, therefore, for clinicians to have the skill to design 'social skills packages' for their clients. Even in group programmes flexibility is necessary. Although the group will follow essentially the same treatment plan, some members are able to skip steps that others require; some need intervening steps that others do not.

The assessment should be tied as closely to the intervention as possible. The desired outcomes of intervention should be reflected in the content of the assessment instruments. The instruments should include skills or concepts organized according to the putative components of the training. To use this approach effectively, we need to know what the goals of the intervention are.

Some therapists use batteries of psychological tests which may be useful for purposes of research or record keeping. However, we do not believe that extensive testing is necessary in the daily practice of therapy for speech disordered clients. Assessment should be as brief as possible as extensive assessment adds to the cost of the therapy and should be adequately justified. Consequently, routine testing is not required unless it will facilitate the therapeutic process in a definable manner. Because of the importance of the initial interview, the therapist needs to be especially alert and active to secure and evaluate the necessary information in a relatively short time. The goal is a concise, concentrated but adequate assessment to reach clinically sound decisions on the course of treatment.

Assessment and treatment basically rely on the therapist's ability to pinpoint the relevant factors that led to the development and maintenance of the undesired behaviour. Treatment has to focus on the most important elements, starting with these and then moving on to secondary factors. The selection of these target behaviours is crucial and relies on the ability to conduct the initial interview skilfully.

It is important to determine whether the client has the ability to understand the concept of communication skills training and is able to co-operate. Teaching approaches will differ considerably for the client who knows what the desirable response should be but who for various reasons fails to perform, as opposed to the client who behaves inappropriately because he does not know what to do.

From the start of therapy clients should acquire self-management skills which will help them maintain their gains after formal treatment ends. It is therefore useful for therapists to explain from the very beginning what they are doing, why they are doing it and how they do it. This not only enhances co-operation of the clients, but helps clients in identifying, analysing and recording the target behaviours themselves, teaching both self-monitoring and self-evaluation. The client would therefore begin to learn these skills by sharing with the therapist in the assessment and evaluation tasks as well as the treatment sessions. The therapist might demonstrate her procedure for keeping data, like using frequency counts for recording discrete behaviours, time sampling or time interval measures for continuous behaviours, or rating scales for more qualitative or subjective measures. The client might practise identification and recording of specific behaviours and compare his scores with the therapist's.

It has become increasingly apparent that changing behaviour within the clinical setting is much less difficult than maintaining it. Therefore assessment has to focus on identifying the maintaining factors in order to deal with them in an effective therapeutic manner.

We will need to incorporate into the assessment procedure not only the prospective client, but also 'significant others'. This is most important for the treatment of children. Their behaviour is powerfully influenced by the environment in general and by their parents in particular. For treatment to be effective, parents have to be involved from the outset. The parents' educational goals and reinforcement systems in operation will help to determine which incentives to use in therapy, transfer and maintenance. Social skills are very situation-specific. Measurement reliability will be enhanced when observing the clients interacting with their family and peers. This is particularly important, as we know from clinical experience that there is little agreement between parents, teachers and children when rating the quality of social behaviour.

Assessment can help determine whether it is a new behaviour that should be taught or whether the environment will have to be modified in some way to help reinforce behaviour that is known but not used.

All social skills input needs to take into account the environment of the clients and the social behaviour of their peers. What is socially acceptable for one group of people is unacceptable for another. For example, eye-contact, which is encouraged in Western society, is not always acceptable in certain ethnic groups. Thus, the therapist should have a clear understanding of the goals in therapy and should ensure that these are realistic.

When assessing stroke patients or clients with severe neurological disorders, it is important for therapists to get an idea of their client's premorbid social functioning as this should be used as a yardstick for judging the level of social behaviour at which therapy can be aimed. Additionally, it is necessary to gain information on the person's past as well as current social relationships and how the neurological deficit is affecting communication.

What situations are most difficult for the client and the carer/spouse? Is the client aware of the problems? Is his performance adequate, if not, is it due to lack of speech and language ability, poor self-expression, or could it be due to severe emotional disturbance? Does the client have a clear idea of what he wants? Does the client realistically appraise his situation and level of functioning?

Deciding whether group or individual training would be most appropriate will depend on the skills of the child or adult. Many speech and language impaired clients might benefit from individual therapy for a set number of sessions prior to being placed in a group.

The interview is augmented by information from the client's family and/or colleagues, and questionnaires. These sources of information help to select the target behaviours for treatment. These behaviours may already exist in the client's repertoire, which means that the therapist is looking to increase their frequency of occurrence, or to reduce or eliminate them. For other clients the desired behaviour may not exist in their repertoire and may have to be built through shaping and successive approximation techniques.

As the initial interview draws to an end, the therapist should try to synthesize the information and observations. At least in a tentative way, the therapist will attempt to evaluate the individual as a prospective member of her next social skills group and in doing so will have weighed the positive, negative, and questionable features and viewed them in terms of some formulation about therapy. If the diagnostic appraisal is unclear, then additional assessment, consultation or referral needs to be considered. When the therapist has decided positively to accept that person for therapy, then the final part of the interview is directed towards orienting the prospective client to the therapy that is to follow.

Beyond the initial assessment it is fruitful to establish a continuous simple outcome evaluation process that will provide relevant measures of progress. This will determine when a client has mastered a particular set of behaviours and the next step can be implemented? Additionally, it gives the therapist information about the quality of her treatment programme. Continuing evaluation easily identifies incorrect steps which can then be rectified.

These measures should be regularly implemented, not only throughout the acquisition, but also during the transfer, generalization, maintenance and follow-up phases of therapy.

Assessment Procedures

There are many ways of assessing patients, such as sociometric questionnaires, observation and recording of performance on video or tape recorder, teacher, parent or carer questionnaires, rating scales including self-rating and peer rating, interview by speech therapist, role play, and physiological measures. There is no specific set of assessments that are applicable to all clients, and therapists will need to make their own objective judgements in many instances. We outline some assessment procedures that can be used with a variety of speech and language disorders.

Clinical Interview

The clinical interview is the traditional method of assessing social skills. The interview takes place on the assumption that the client is potentially the richest source of information about himself. Where clients are speech or language handicapped, an oral interview might present difficulties. There are a wide range of assessment interviews, from the sophisticated and lengthy as designed for adolescent stammerers (Rustin, Cook and Spence, 1995), to the short and simple designed for use with adult learning disabled clients (Hitchings and Spence, 1991; Kelly, 1996).

General Steps for Assessment

General steps for assessment should include the following.

- Explanation of purpose of assessment.
- Identification of range of problems.
- Selection of main problems, establishment of priorities.
- Identification of present problem behaviour (antecedents, consequences, secondary gains, previous attempts at solving the problem).
- Identification of coping skills.
- Clients' perception of problem (intensity).

- What is the major problem? Are there secondary problems — behavioural/cognitive/affective/physiological, (What? When? Where? How often? With whom? How distressing? How disruptive?).
- What are the relevant situations (context)?
- What is the time course?
- What are the predisposing factors?
- What skills are available? What is missing?
- Is there evidence of avoidance behaviour?
- Are the necessary skills there but is it not possible to put them into practice because of negative thoughts, anxiety or depression (mood/mental state)?
- What are the expectations from therapy?
- What is the psychosocial situation (family, social relationships, hobbies/interests)?

Having defined the problem, the next step will be to select and define goals with the client.

- What would you like to change about yourself?
- If this change is accomplished, how would things be different (for yourself, for others)?
- How feasible is this change (advantages, risks)?
- What resources can be used (skills/knowledge, people) to attain the goal?
- What obstacles (people, feelings, ideas, situations) might interfere with goal attainment?
- How could you monitor and review progress towards the goal?

It is also important to establish the precedent and consequent factors that might control certain undesirable behaviours. Observation of the client's interaction during the interview has the unique advantage of providing contextual and qualitative elaboration of events that are, or were, important to the individual. They allow the therapist to gain an overall picture of the history of interpersonal activity and choose and elaborate on those categories of social skills that are relevant to a client and explore them in depth (e.g. social activities, reaction to anger/frustration, interpersonal behaviour patterns in the family). Self-report inventories might be used as guides during the interview to elaborate on specific points.

Whilst there are many advantages to interviews being unstructured and flexible, it is important for therapists to be aware of pitfalls, such as bias, making assumptions based on misinformation from other sources, omitting questions that may be relevant, etc. Having completed an interview, the therapist will be able to generate hypotheses that will structure the continuing assessment process.

Observation

This method of assessment is valuable and the therapist will need to have developed her own observational skills to a high level. It is useful for the therapist to arrange to observe the client in his own environment if possible so that note can be taken of how the client's behaviour changes within settings outside the clinic. Therapists should also be aware of how social interaction changes when the patient's speech deteriorates.

Walker *et al.* (1983), in their programme, describe a format for making direct observational measures of the amount of time a child participates socially with peers in the playground, in a structured activity and in the classroom. This information, used in conjunction with a checklist, provides a comprehensive picture of the child's classroom and social adjustments. There is also a 'placement test' included in the programme which identifies the specific skills in the curriculum that the child should be taught. All of these assessments rely on the teacher's, therapist's and helper's direct observations of the child in the school setting.

Observation in the natural environment should be directed towards defined social behaviours. There are various ways of recording events, e.g. tally counters to count frequency of the occurrence or non-occurrence of a behaviour during a set time interval. To lessen the reactive effects of observation techniques, this should be done as unobtrusively as possible.

Rinaldi's (1992, 1993) social use of language programmes were designed for secondary school/young adult learning disabled people and primary and pre-school children, respectively. Both these programmes offer an assessment profile based on the observations of teachers, therapists, assistants, etc. over a period of two to three weeks. The areas covered in assessment are listening, turn-taking, speaking and understanding.

Rustin, Botterill and Kelman (1996) developed an interaction profile that looked at a wide range of social interactions that could be evaluated using a six-minute videotaped sample of a parent playing with his or her child (see Figure 8.1). This was developed initially for use with dysfluent children and has been adapted for use with children with delayed speech and language development.

There are three main approaches to observation:

1. *In vivo* observation, which is most desirable but least practical.
2. Naturalistic interactions, using structured or staged interactions which are intended to parallel *in vivo* encounters. In these cases, trained confederates are used to interact with the subjects. The realism of the interaction depends on the acting abilities of the confederate.

Non-verbal		Verbal
	Directiveness	
	Following child's lead	
Listening		Turn-taking
		Balance of conversation
		Interrupting
	Giving time to respond	
	Pausing	
Gaining child's attention		Rate
		Intelligibility
Observation		Volume
Eye contact with child		Fluency
Shared focus of attention		Prosody
Facial expression		Complexity: syntactic
Animation		semantic
Intrigue		Semantic contingency
Touch		
Gesture		Initiation
		• Questions/requests
		• Imperatives
Position		• Comments
• level		• Other
• mobility		
• orientation		Commenting
• proximity		Responding
		Repetition
Manner		Rephrasing
• warmth		Maintaining topic
• attachment	Reinforcement	Repair
	Conflict management	
	Choice of activity	
	Response to speech	
	difficulty	

Figure 8.1: Interaction profile

3. Role play: An interpersonal vignette is described to the subjects, a role model (confederate) utters a prompt line and the subject responds, thereby setting the interaction sequence in motion. This can be repeated with different situations from all areas of specific interest to the client. Sufficient data must be collected to establish that the rate of a behaviour is stable. There are standardized role play procedures that could be used but we feel that the trainers/therapists themselves would have to choose the appropriate situations in terms

of the goals that are to be achieved. The length of time, the format, the level of structure, the type of response required, the instructions and scoring of measures will need to be adapted to the specific client group.

The disadvantages of role play are that its external and social validity is doubtful and there is also a lack of normative data. However, together with other methods of assessment, it might indicate some of the client's strengths and weaknesses. We feel that its advantages far outweigh the disadvantages in that it is possible to present to the client a wide range of potentially relevant situations that cannot easily be replicated in the natural environment.

It is difficult reliably to assess affective responses; however, self-reports, observation of clients' body language and behaviours that are interpreted as outward signs of inner reactions are most commonly used.

Rinaldi (1993) included in her assessment process self/other aware-ness interview. The child is asked to make statements about himself as a person, his appearance, interests, strengths, weaknesses and feelings. The child is then asked to do the same with some of his friends.

Assessing Cognitions

Cognitive skills are important in order to become more effective in solving problems and developing general social skills. It is necessary to be able to 'perceive' and to 'translate': to judge accurately the behaviour of others and the nature of the interaction, and to interpret correctly the feedback from others in judging one's own performance (perception). The therapist will need to assess clients' ability to make inferences about other people's thoughts and feelings as well as their degree of empathy, which is the ability to share the feelings of others, and, following from this, the ability to generate a range of alternative responses, to predict likely outcomes and select accordingly, and plan the component responses to carry out the response selected.

Social skills training is designed to enhance observational, perform-ance, and cognitive skills related to effective social behaviours in partic-ular situations. Deficiencies in skilled behaviour may involve an inappropriate goal, inaccurate perception or translation, or deficient performance, as well as a variety of other factors, including anxiety in social situations.

The basic rationale of assessment is that thoughts, feelings and atti-tudes influence behaviour, and that behaviour can influence thoughts, feelings and attitudes. The assessment therefore has to blend the more empirical and specific approach to behaviour with the more abstract and harder to objectify aspects of inner processes. Therefore, assessment should aim at studying the relationships among covert phenomena and their relationship to patterns of behaviour and expressions of emotion. What are the channels between attributions, expectations, current concerns, self-statements, images, beliefs, etc. to expressed behaviour? The central principle of cognitive–behavioural assessment is that the ways in which an individual behaves are determined by immediate situations, and the individual's interpretations of these. This 'view of the world' becomes the major focus of the assessment, with an emphasis on specific problems.

Although most of the assessment takes place in the initial sessions, the assessment process continues throughout treatment. The following factors should be determined in the assessment of cognitive behaviours:

1. Does the client have a cognitive understanding of the behaviours being taught?
2. Are there faulty cognitions that interfere with desirable social behaviour?
3. Is there a lack of problem solving strategies?

In most cases irrational beliefs are assessed during the clinical interview. Unless interviewer and client share a similar cognitive view of psychological problems and speak in a common cognitively based language, the therapist has to begin this part of the interview with several 'educational statements' whereby the interviewer encourages clients to examine their difficulties in a cognitive light. In this part of the interview there is already some overlap between assessment and treatment. The therapist not only identifies the dysfunctional belief system in the client's presenting symptoms but also shares this information with the client, in effect, the therapist tells the client what his rational/irrational beliefs are.

The assessment takes place in an analogue format: real-life events are described and the clients' reactions are recorded, or a selection of possible reactions is presented to the clients and they must choose the one which they feel is appropriate. An important part of assessing cognitions is the search for maladaptive self-statements, assumptions and beliefs, perfectionistic thinking and inaccurate attributions where clients fail to accept responsibility for their behaviour but attribute their actions to external factors.

Several techniques may facilitate the within-interview identification of irrational beliefs. Clients would describe typical situations in which their speech impairment causes problems and situations in which they are upset or anxious, they are then asked to explore related thoughts, attitudes, and assumptions. Their content will indicate the irrational belief responsible for the distress. Clients' statements that refer to specific emotions are useful for assessing irrational beliefs since rational emotive theory suggests that particular emotional consequences follow from adherence to certain irrational beliefs. For example, clients may report feeling depressed over a situation in which they failed with their speech. When questioned further this could be the result of an irrational belief that their speech must be perfect in order to be acceptable.

Clinical experience shows that cognitive behavioural techniques seem to be most attractive and work best with an educated and articulate clientele. Even if behavioural tasks are assigned, the emphasis is clearly on ideas and thoughts. Individuals with more limited education and intellectual resources might not be as responsive.

Video Recording/Rating Scales

Use of video recordings for the assessment of social ability is a well-recognized method and is of particular value for the speech and language impaired as it records their speech and language ability as well as their social interaction. A two- to five-minute videotape recording should be made of the client interacting with:

1. The therapist.
2. Parent, spouse or carer.
3. Peers.

The therapist could then make a list of difficulties that might be encountered by a patient with a specific disorder and rate them accordingly (see Figure 8.2).

Skills	Rating Scale				
	Poor 1 →	2 →	3 →	4 →	Good 5 →
Eye-contact					
Observation					
Listening					
Turn-taking					
Excessive body movements					
Attention and concentration					
Conversational repair					
Initiation/termination of conversation					
Facial expression					
Posture					
Gesture					
Praise/reinforcement					
Prosody					
Tension/irritability					

Figure 8.2: Rating of difficulties encountered

The scale can be checked with a colleague to gain inter-rater reliability and should be discussed where appropriate with the client. He should then be helped to fill in a similar rating scale, following observation of the video. Thus, agreement regarding any changes that might need to be made with respect to social interaction can be reached before remediation is incorporated into the speech therapy intervention. It is often helpful to discuss and use the rating scale with carers. The video interaction also enables the therapist to observe what reinforcement the carers and peers give to the patient and whether it needs to be changed in a way that will be helpful for the patient. Where possible, it will be of value if videos can be made *in situ* in the patient's environment.

Rating scales are an extremely useful measure of change, even though their external reliability is low.

Checklists

These might be filled in by individuals associated with the client, i.e. parents, teachers, nurses, etc. Their social validity is normally quite high if the raters are well trained. If they are not, there could be inconsistencies caused by personal bias or carelessness. However, they are easy to administer and analyse and can give valuable information in conjunction with other assessment techniques (see Figures 8.3 and 8.4).

Self-report

Self-reports have an intermediary role between checklists and behavioural observation. The client is instructed to observe on-going events systematically, thereby helping to reduce subjective distortions, errors of recall, etc. It has been found that self-reports are sensitive to change and could therefore be used to assess treatment changes during treatment. They might be useful in evaluating the effectiveness of training (see Figures 8.5 and 8.6).

Self-observation

Self-observation is a form of self-exploration. It helps clients and therapists to define the problem more clearly and to formulate therapeutic possibilities.

The process of self-observation allows clients to become more aware of facts, thoughts and emotions which have been previously overlooked, thereby making it easier to define the problem and formulate therapeutic priorities. A client may realize that there are specific conditions under which undesirable behaviour occurs, or the client redefines the original problem as he review the facts.

	Good 1	Adequate 2	Seldom 3	Poor 4
Name of client: _____ Date: _____				
Assessor: _____				
Foundation Skills				
Makes eye contact when speaking	1	2	3	4
Makes eye contact when listening	1	2	3	4
Able to observe others	1	2	3	4
Grooming	1	2	3	4
Facial expression	1	2	3	4
Gesture	1	2	3	4
Posture	1	2	3	4
Proximity	1	2	3	4
Ability to listen to others	1	2	3	4
Tone/volume of voice	1	2	3	4
Able to remember what is being said to them	1	2	3	4
Affective Skills				
Identification of own feeling	1	2	3	4
Recognizing feelings of others — express appreciation	1	2	3	4
Able to talk about self appropriately	1	2	3	4
Shares appropriately	1	2	3	4
Express affection	1	2	3	4
Express negative feeling	1	2	3	4
Express positive feeling	1	2	3	4
Interaction Skills				
Starting conversation	1	2	3	4
Asking questions	1	2	3	4
Ability to respond to questioning	1	2	3	4
Maintain a conversation	1	2	3	4
Repair breakdown of conversation	1	2	3	4
End a conversation	1	2	3	4
Makes positive comments to others (compliments)	1	2	3	4
Offers to assist others	1	2	3	4
Responds to others	1	2	3	4
Co-operates with others	1	2	3	4
Complies with reasonable requests	1	2	3	4
Takes turns in conversation	1	2	3	4
Cognitive Skills				
Addresses others appropriately	1	2	3	4
Follows group rules	1	2	3	4
Participates in group activities	1	2	3	4
Asks to stop actions	1	2	3	4
Asks for reasons	1	2	3	4
Tells reasons	1	2	3	4
Complains	1	2	3	4
Responds appropriately to complaints	1	2	3	4
Makes suggestions	1	2	3	4

Figure 8.3: Checklist for communication skills rating

Name of Client: _____   Date:
Name of Assessor: _____
Enter skills to be assessed in first column

SKILL	Date: 1 2 3	Date: 1 2 3	Date: 1 2 3	Date: 1 2 3

Rating Guide: 1. Client does not exhibit skill
               2. Client exhibits skill occasionally but less than acceptable.
               3. Client exhibits skill at acceptable level

Figure 8.4: Professionals' Assessment Rating Scale

Descriptions of exactly what is done, said, thought and felt in relevant situations should be obtained. It might be useful to complement clients' reports with data from other sources, because clients might not be able to identify important aspects of their social behaviour or they may misrepresent the reactions of others.

Physiological Assessment

Anxiety is very often cited as an important variable in social skills dysfunction. It has been well documented that stress reactions can manifest themselves in any of three response systems: motoric, cognitive and physiological. Therefore, it is generally recommended that behavioural assessment should encompass these three channels. Despite this, the relevance of physiological assessment for the evaluation of social skills is uncertain. There is no clear picture of the relationship of autonomic arousal to social skills. However, for some individuals, biofeedback methods might be beneficial, especially in those cases where receptivity of internal cues is lacking. Physiological processes may be monitored indirectly by asking a socially phobic client to rate the amount perspired in social situations.

Although psychological measurement has been used extensively in research, its use in routine clinical practice is limited by the cost, practicality and availability of equipment.

Name: _____

Place a ring round the numbers on the right according to how good you think you are at each communication task. Use the numbers as follows:

1 = This is a task I am *ALWAYS* good at
2 = This is a task I am *USUALLY* good at
3 = This is a task I am *SOMETIMES* good at
4 = This is a task I am *NEVER* good at

1.	Starting a conversation	1	2	3	4
2.	Listening to people	1	2	3	4
3.	Asking questions	1	2	3	4
4.	Keeping a conversation going	1	2	3	4
5.	Holding a telephone conversation	1	2	3	4
6.	Saying 'thank you'	1	2	3	4
7.	Talking to people in authority	1	2	3	4
8.	Talking about myself	1	2	3	4
9.	Apologizing when I have done something wrong	1	2	3	4
10.	Complimenting others	1	2	3	4
11.	Talking to members of the opposite sex	1	2	3	4
12.	Ending a conversation	1	2	3	4
13.	Asking for favours	1	2	3	4
14.	Sharing sympathy when people tell me their problems	1	2	3	4
15.	Concentrating on the other person when I am talking to them	1	2	3	4
16.	Talking to strangers	1	2	3	4
17.	Talking to people I don't know well	1	2	3	4
18.	Talking to my friends	1	2	3	4
19.	Talking to my family	1	2	3	4
20.	Asking someone to stop doing something I don't like	1	2	3	4

Figure 8.5: Example of a self-report form

Conclusions

A study by Marzillier and Winter (1978) highlights the importance of assessment and the need for careful behavioural analysis prior to choosing a treatment strategy. They used social skills training in the treatment of four psychiatric outpatients with social difficulties. Three out of four cases improved and one reacted adversely to treatment and dropped out. The patient's reluctance to pursue treatment further was not due to the ineffectiveness of the training programme but because therapeutic procedures evoked excessive anxiety which could not be adequately controlled. It was also noted that the behavioural changes that occurred in the clinical setting were not necessarily generalized. Therefore, initial assessment alone is not sufficient. We need to check repeatedly that our procedures are not only effective in behavioural

terms but that they do not evoke destructive emotions, such as high
levels of anxiety.

In conclusion, social skills assessment should encompass a measurement of both physical and psychological components. We need to be aware
of limitations, either genetic or cultural, including physical and/or mental
deficits. The assessment strategy should be practical and will vary according
to available resources. However, we should like to stress the importance of
assessment procedures not only in helping the therapist analyse the
client's problems but also in knowing how best to remediate them.

Name: Date:					
Please rate your skills in the following areas:	never good	rarely good	sometimes good	often good	always good
1. Looking at people when I'm talking to them and they are talking to me					
2. Listening to what other people have to say					
3. Starting a conversation					
4. Taking turns in a conversation					
5. Asking questions					
6. Answering questions					
7. Maintaining an appropriate distance between myself and others when I'm talking					
8. Praising other people					
9. Disagreeing with others					
10. Agreeing with others					
11. Finding solutions to problems					
12. Talking at the right speed (not too fast, not too slow)					
			TOTAL		

Figure 8.6: Social communication skills. Self-rating scale

Concluding Remarks

The review of the literature and our clinical experience have shown that social skills training is a valuable tool to help clients adapt to the ever changing demands in our society. Social skills are important in many respects, in leading a satisfactory personal life as well as being successful at work. We are aware that this book is only a small step towards differential treatment for the communicatively handicapped. However, the gain in knowledge will be greater and the benefit for our clients more substantial if we succeed in helping therapists to develop their own ideas in relation to social skills training in the treatment of speech and language impaired clients. The role of the therapist is crucial as social skills training is not the simple application of research findings to everyday social problems.

We hope that by helping the speech and language impaired to develop their social skills, they will be able to lead a fuller life within the restrictions of their disability.

Part II

Chapter 9
Exercises

Introduction

Having established the need for social skills training in a particular client group, and assessed the abilities of the individual, the therapist will decide on the skill level at which to begin the training programme. For easy reference the individual skills have been grouped into four categories: foundation skills, interaction skills, affective skills and cognitive skills. The key at the top of each exercise (see pp. 152 – 264) shows which skills the particular exercise is aimed at and the footnote shows in bold type the client group for which the exercise is most relevant. The tables (pp. 113 – 151) show which exercises to use for which client group.

Foundation Skills

Foundation skills include:

- Gelling.
- Observation.
- Eye-contact.
- Posture.
- Presentation/grooming.
- Facial expression.
- Gesture.
- Space/proximity.
- Listening (basic).
- Volume, prosody, tone, pitch.
- Relaxation.
- Touch.
- Memory.

Foundation skills are basic skills and are fundamental to the development of more sophisticated social interactions. Thus clients need to be well versed in these skills, as they will facilitate the acquisition of more complex skills at a later stage. For some client groups, for example those with severe learning disability, training programmes might be exclusively directed at this level, whilst for other groups, such as adolescent stutterers, selected skills may be targeted from all four categories.

Interaction Skills

Interaction skills include:

- Greetings.
- Initiating/asking questions.
- Listening/reflecting back, responding.
- Answering questions/responding.
- Reinforcement.
- Topic maintenance/repair of conversations.
- Termination.
- Co-operating.
- Turn-taking, breaking in, interrupting.

The skills within this category are more complex than foundation skills as they often require the combination of two or more skills being in operation at the same time, for example topic maintenance may require listening, observation, turn-taking, facial expression, gesture, etc. A higher level of verbal language skills is necessary for the exercises within this category and therefore the therapist will need to select those skills that are within the linguistic competence of the client and focus on the pragmatic and functional aspects of language.

Affective Skills

Affective skills include:

- Identification of feelings.
- Recognizing own feelings.
- Recognizing feelings of others.
- Trust.
- Disclosures.

The skills within this category help clients understand the influence of thoughts and feelings on social behaviour and its important role in developing relationships. A range of feelings are identified, described and discussed. Clients explore their own feelings and discover ways of expressing these verbally and non-verbally. In addition, the exercises help them to interpret the verbal and non-verbal signals of others, thus enhancing their ability to interact more effectively.

Cognitive Skills

Cognitive skills include:

- Social perception.
- Problem solving.
- Self-instruction.
- Self-monitoring, evaluation and reinforcement.
- Praise/reinforcement.
- Negotiating.
- Assertion.

These are the most complex skills requiring the employment of many of the skills in the previous categories. These skills help participants explore the role they play in social settings, the choices they have and the process of decision making. Clients are given the opportunity to practise these skills and experiment with alternatives in the safe environment of the clinic before trying them out in the real world.

Using the Exercises

The exercises described in this book are useful tools in the process of sensitizing clients towards the usefulness of a particular skill. They provide an easy relaxed way of experimenting with new behaviours out of their normal context. For example, a group of children need to learn about eye-contact, so they can begin a session with exercise 79: Eye-swap chairs, an exercise that is fun but requires them to give each other eye-contact as a cue to swapping chairs. A discussion after the exercise can be led to isolate the skill necessary to be successful in this game and then why it might also enhance good communication.

In this way there are exercises that will apply to all the skills in the four categories described. Many of the exercises can be used in a variety of ways to teach a number of different skills according to the needs of the clients. They are cross-referenced for the category of skills that may be taught and also the client group for whom they might be appropriate as shown in Chart for Practical Activities (p.229).

Skills and Exercise Analysis

All exercises are displayed in the Appendix p.115 according to their application to the different speech and language disorders.

To use the table identify skills on which you wish to focus and find corresponding exercise numbers.

Running these exercises in a group also involves the participants in learning skills related to their roles in a social group, such as sharing, teamwork, leadership, co-operation, following rules, and managing 'losing and winning'.

These exercises are highly versatile and when used appropriately are motivating and fun for both children and adults. In the relaxed atmosphere that is created clients are more able to 'let go' and experiment with new things and be more tolerant of their own and others' mistakes.

Exercises are of particular value with more difficult skills as they enable the therapist to approach the final goals systematically, starting off with easy tasks then progressing to more difficult ones. Because of their distance from real life, exercises also provide the opportunity to try out new behaviours and make mistakes without negative consequences.

Running the Exercises

Having chosen the appropriate exercises for the social skill that is to be worked on, instructions should be given clearly. It might be necessary to repeat them to ensure that everyone has understood what is required of them. This will avoid clients getting confused, which could interrupt the flow of the exercise. Having completed the exercise there should be a period of discussion related to its purposes. This stage is of great importance and should not be rushed as it can be a significant part of the individual or group's personal experience and it gives an opportunity to further self-awareness. Participants will benefit from the opportunity to explore their own feelings and thoughts following an exercise, and each member of the group should be given the time to express his views. Where appropriate, the discussion might include the implications the exercise has in relation to their everyday life.

Video Recording

For many clients, building self-awareness and self-monitoring skills are the key to transfer and maintenance of their new behaviours. Judicious use of video recordings has a vital role in helping clients to develop these difficult but essential skills. Participants can be helped to identify their own strengths and make decisions about the behaviours that they wish to change or modify. This form of experimental learning is very powerful and can enable clients with a wide variety of difficulties to make changes and improve their social interaction skills.

Any programme for speech and language impaired clients should consider including the five core skills outlined below.

Observation

Effective communication requires the understanding of non-verbal signals such as body language, appearance and proximity as well as verbal signals. Failure to respond to these non-verbal signals may cause misunderstandings and inappropriate responses. Clients who have poor eye-contact or do not make use of non-verbal information will be more likely to 'misinterpret' a situation and give an incorrect response. It is usual for a speaker to break eye-contact when thinking, whereas the listener should give more continual eye gaze. Hargie *et al.* (1981) list the following non-verbal behaviours which aid successful communication:

- Nods of head.
- Appropriate smiles.
- Direct eye-contact.
- Mirroring facial expressions.
- Adopting an attentive posture.

Many clients with speech and language impairment have poor observation skills due to developmental or acquired conditions and need to improve this basic skill.

Listening

Being a good listener is perhaps the most important skill for successful communication but the one that many speech and language impaired clients have great difficulty in acquiring. Listening is complex and involves many skills both verbal and non-verbal, such as attention, hearing, understanding and memory, eye-contact, and body language. Furthermore, it is important for listeners to learn how to demonstrate to the speaker that they are listening through appropriate use of eye-contact, body posture, reinforcement (smiling, head nods, etc.) and turn-taking. Parents, teachers and carers may become focused on encouraging the expressive skills of the speech and language impaired to the detriment of the listener role. Communication is a process of which listening skills are an essential component. If these are neglected the successful functioning of this process is put at risk.

Turn-Taking

Both observation and listening skills are fundamental to the ability to take turns in conversation. Speech and language impaired patients often have difficulty in breaking into a conversation as well as relinquishing their turn. Taking turns in speaking and listening is important in developing and maintaining a conversation. Non-verbal signals are given by eye-contact and inflection of voice to indicate when someone is ready to complete their turn. The speaker may also respond to the non-verbal signals of the listener, who will indicate through eye-contact, facial expression and posture that they would like a 'turn'. Turn-taking operates by mutual agreement and does not necessarily require equal contributions from both parties. Successful turn-taking involves good timing and pausing, thus avoiding interruptions and long silences. It is often important for the speech and language impaired to learn to tolerate silent pauses in a conversation and not to become anxious, thus exacerbating their speech difficulty.

Reinforcement

This skill at the simplest level involves basic non-verbal responses such as eye-contact, smiling and nods of the head, or verbal encouragement such as 'really'. 'which', 'mm'. However, at its most complex, reinforcement is a highly sophisticated skill that can be responsible for profoundly changing the behaviour of others, and individuals' view of themselves. Reinforcement used judiciously in an interaction encourages conversation, demonstrates an interest in the ideas, thoughts and feelings expressed by others, and creates a warm and sympathetic environment, making it more enjoyable and rewarding for those involved. Those who have mastered the basic-level skills should be encouraged to tackle the more sophisticated verbal skills involved in acknowledging, confirming, encouraging, praise (giving and receiving), and support. Care must be taken on the part of clinicians and clients to use reinforcement immediately, whilst also varying the content in relation to the context.

Problem Solving

This skill requires participants to generate alternatives in a situation and then make a choice. The level of complexity will vary from, 'what items of clothing to wear in the morning', to more complex issues such as, 'how to deal with teasing at school', 'how to ask the boss for a rise', etc. The importance of problem solving, however, is in encouraging independent decision-making. It provides the opportunity for participants to experience the process by being creative and experimenting in a safe and supportive environment. As clients become more practised and familiar with problem solving, they become more confident, self-determined, and assertive. These skills will be invaluable to them as they learn to manage in the 'real world' outside the clinic.

Generalization of exercises will be enhanced by encouraging risk taking and humour on the part of clients. The therapist should establish well-defined limits and rules as well as goals and objectives which should be clearly understood. Immediate feedback should always be provided regarding the results of the exercises. Therapists will find it helpful to familiarize themselves thoroughly with the exercises prior to using them with clients.

Practical Activities

Foundation Skills
Eye-contact
posture
facial expression
gesture
space/proximity
listening (basic)
volume, prosody, tone, pitch
memory

Interaction Skills
listening
termination
turn-taking

Affective Skills
disclosures

Cognitive Skills
self-monitoring evaluation and
    reinforcement

---

1. THE LISTENING EXERCISE

The group is divided into sub-groups of three people. Within each triad, there should be a speaker, a listener and an observer. The speaker and listener should sit opposite each other whilst the observer is seated at right angles to them:

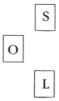

The therapist instructs the speaker to give a short simple account of an event which *actually* happened to them. The listener should listen to what is said, then repeat back the narrative as accurately as possible to the speaker. The observer is to listen to both accounts and then comment on the listener's performance. The exercise is repeated until each person had adopted each role. This exercise may lead to a full discussion on listening.

Modification
To simplify:
• Specify a limited number of sentences to be included in the narrative.

VOICE	LARYNGECTOMY	PHYSICAL DISABILITY	PHONOLOGICAL IMPAIRMENT	MENTAL ILLNESS	HEARING IMPAIRMENT
STUTTER	DYSPHASIA	LEARNING DISABILITY	DYSPRAXIA DYSARTHRIA	ELDERLY	LANGUAGE IMPAIRMENT

Foundation Skills	**Interaction Skills**
gelling	initiation/asking questions
observation	answering questions/responding
eye-contact	co-operating
space/proximity	turn-taking
listening (basic)	
touch	
memory	

Affective Skills	**Cognitive Skills**
	problem solving
	assertion

2. FAMOUS NAMES

Labels are prepared. The name of a famous person is written on each label, e.g. sportsperson, film star. The labels are attached to each group member's back without them seeing what is written on it. The members of the group are then instructed to move around and ask each other questions to find out who they are meant to be. The questions should be closed and only require a 'yes' or 'no' response, e.g. 'Am I a man?' Do I play sport?'. When everyone has discovered who they are, the group reassembles to discuss any difficulties or problems that they encountered.

Modifications

To simplify:
- Instead of famous people, use common objects, e.g. book, apple, pencil.
- Do not restrict questions to 'yes' or 'no' answers but allow open questions to be used, e.g. 'what am I used for?'.

Non-readers:
- Use a photograph or picture of person or object.

Limited mobility:
- Divide the group into pairs, who then question one another.

VOICE	LARYNGECTOMY	**PHYSICAL DISABILITY**	**PHONOLOGICAL IMPAIRMENT**	**MENTAL ILLNESS**	**HEARING IMPAIRMENT**
STUTTER	**DYSPHASIA**	**LEARNING DISABILITY**	**DYSPRAXIA DYSARTHRIA**	**ELDERLY**	**LANGUAGE IMPAIRMENT**

Foundation Skills   **Interaction Skills**
gelling
observation
eye-contact
space/proximity
memory

Affective Skills   **Cognitive Skills**
                                       problem solving

3. WHO IS MISSING?

Group members should be randomly seated around the room either on chairs or on the floor. One person is selected to observe how everyone is placed and then leaves the room. Meanwhile, within the room, everyone changes places except one person, who is to hide. The observer then returns to the room and is allowed 30 seconds to decide who is missing.

Modifications
To simplify:
* Limit the number of people in the exercise.

Limited mobility:
* Helpers move members around.
* The therapist and helpers demonstrate the exercise.
* Arrange the seating more formally, e.g. in a line.

VOICE	LARYNGECTOMY	PHYSICAL DISABILITY	PHONOLOGICAL IMPAIRMENT	MENTAL ILLNESS	HEARING IMPAIRMENT
STUTTER	DYSPHASIA	LEARNING DISABILITY	DYSPRAXIA DYSARTHRIA	ELDERLY	LANGUAGE IMPAIRMENT

Foundation Skills   **Interaction Skills**
gelling   co-operating
eye-contact   breaking in
lisening (basic)
volume
memory

Affective Skills   **Cognitive Skills**
                                 assertion

---

4. LISTEN FOR YOUR PARTNER

Cards are prepared on which are written common paired items, e.g. salt and pepper. Each half of a pair is written on a separate card. The group stands in a circle and a card is given to each member. Everyone is then instructed to call out simultaneously the word on their card in order to find their partner.

Modifications
To simplify:
Non-readers:
• Use pictures of common paired items.

Non-verbal:
• Members hold up pictures, find their pair and stand together.

VOICE	LARYNGECTOMY	**PHYSICAL DISABILITY**	**PHONOLOGICAL IMPAIRMENT**	MENTAL ILLNESS	**HEARING IMPAIRMENT**
STUTTER	DYSPHASIA	**LEARNING DISABILITY**	DYSPRAXIA DYSARTHRIA	ELDERLY	**LANGUAGE IMPAIRMENT**

Foundation Skills
gelling
observation
eye-contact
posture
facial expression
gesture

Interaction Skills
asking questions
answering questions/responding
co-operating
turn-taking

Affective Skills
identification of feelings
recognizing own feelings
recognizing feelings of others

Cognitive Skills
self-instruction
self-monitoring evaluation and
reinforcement

5. EMOTIONAL BODY PARTS

Two sets of cards are prepared. One set should have various body parts written on the cards whilst the second set should have different emotions. The group is divided into pairs and each person is given two cards — one from each set. Each member will take it in turns to express to their partner the emotion on one card with the body part on the other card, e.g. happy feet, angry hand. Their partner should try to guess the emotion.

Modifications
To simplify:
• Use only one set of cards and specify the body part to be used.

Non-reader:
• Present a picture of the body part and the emotion.

Limited mobility:
• Only suggest body parts which have good function.

VOICE	LARYNGECTOMY	PHYSICAL DISABILITY	PHONOLOGICAL IMPAIRMENT	MENTAL ILLNESS	HEARING IMPAIRMENT
STUTTER	DYSPHASIA	LEARNING DISABILITY	DYSPRAXIA DYSARTHRIA	ELDERLY	LANGUAGE IMPAIRMENT

Foundation Skills	Interaction Skills
observation	
posture	
listening (basic)	
relaxation	

Affective Skills	Cognitive Skills

6. SNOWMEN

The group are instructed to stand like snowmen — frozen stiff, tightly packed ice, out in the cold. The group leader then describes the sun coming out and warming the snowmen, so they begin to melt, getting wet and dripping, then thawing and melting into a puddle. The snowmen may start to freeze again because it is night-time, thus contrasting the two states. (Music may be used to accompany this exercise.)

Modifications

To simplify:

- Demonstrate by melting an ice cube over a heat source.
- Therapist may demonstrate the action of a freezing snowman and a melting one.

VOICE	LARYNGECTOMY	**PHYSICAL DISABILITY**	**PHONOLOGICAL IMPAIRMENT**	MENTAL ILLNESS	**HEARING IMPAIRMENT**
STUTTER	DYSPHASIA	**LEARNING DISABILITY**	DYSPRAXIA DYSARTHRIA	ELDERLY	**LANGUAGE IMPAIRMENT**

Foundation Skills   **Interaction Skills**
gelling
observation
eye-contact
posture
facial expression
space/proximity

Affective Skills   **Cognitive Skills**
recognizing feelings of others   problem solving

7. WHO HAS THE BALL?

The group members stand in a circle and one person leaves the room. The group pass or throw a small ball to one another. When the person outside is ready to come back, they must knock three times and enter as quickly as possible after knocking. The person who has the ball when the knocking starts must try to hide it about their person, and all the other members must try to look as if they have the ball. The person who was outside must guess who has the ball. After each group member has had a turn at discovering who has the ball, the group reassembles to discuss how they discovered who was hiding the ball.

Modifications
Limited verbal comprehension:
* The therapist and helpers demonstrate the exercise.

Limited mobility:
* The helpers move the ball around and assist in hiding it.

VOICE	LARYNGECTOMY	**PHYSICAL DISABILITY**	**PHONOLOGICAL IMPAIRMENT**	MENTAL ILLNESS	**HEARING IMPAIRMENT**
STUTTER	DYSPHASIA	**LEARNING DISABILITY**	DYSPRAXIA DYSARTHRIA	ELDERLY	**LANGUAGE IMPAIRMENT**

Foundation Skills	Interaction Skills
gelling	
observation	
eye-contact	
posture	
space/proximity	
touch	

Affective Skills	Cognitive Skills

8. WINKING PARTNERS

The group is divided into pairs except for one member who is not allocated a partner. The chairs are arranged in a circle. One member of each pair sits on a chair whilst their partner stands behind them, leaving one person standing behind an empty chair. This person winks at a seated person, who then tries to run to the empty chair to form a new partnership before his present partner (behind the chair) stops him by tapping him on the shoulder. This process is repeated a few times, then the group re-forms to discuss the importance of eye contact in successful communication.

Modifications
To simplify:
• The exercise should be demonstrated non-verbally.

Limited mobility:
• Members who are unable to move to a vacant chair should respond to the wink by raising their hand and if they do so before their partner taps them, they can be moved to the vacant place.

VOICE	LARYNGECTOMY	**PHYSICAL DISABILITY**	**PHONOLOGICAL IMPAIRMENT**	**MENTAL ILLNESS**	**HEARING IMPAIRMENT**
STUTTER	DYSPHASIA	**LEARNING DISABILITY**	DYSPRAXIA DYSARTHRIA	ELDERLY	**LANGUAGE IMPAIRMENT**

Foundation Skills
observation
posture
listening (basic)
relaxation

Interaction Skills

Affective Skills

Cognitive Skills

9. TIN SOLDIERS AND RAG DOLLS

Members of the group are instructed to march around the room keeping their bodies stiff and straight, just like tin soldiers or robots. They are then instructed to walk around like limp floppy rag dolls and finally end up in a crumpled heap on the floor. This exercise can be accompanied by appropriate music.

Modifications
To simplify:
• The therapist should demonstrate both postures.
• The therapist can show the group an actual tin soldier or robot and a rag doll, and discuss the differences.

VOICE	LARYNGECTOMY	**PHYSICAL DISABILITY**	**PHONOLOGICAL IMPAIRMENT**	MENTAL ILLNESS	**HEARING IMPAIRMENT**
STUTTER	DYSPHASIA	**LEARNING DISABILITY**	DYSPRAXIA DYSARTHRIA	ELDERLY	**LANGUAGE IMPAIRMENT**

Foundation Skills	**Interaction Skills**
observation	
posture	
listening (basic)	
relaxation	

Affective Skills	**Cognitive Skills**

10. STIFF AND WOBBLY FOODS

The group is instructed to think of different types of food which are stiff or wobbly, e.g.:
- stiff: celery, carrots, twiglets
- wobbly: jelly, custard, yoghurt.

The group leader then calls out one of these foods and the group members pretend to be the food, contrasting the wobbly with the stiff.

Modification
To simplify:
- Present actual foods and encourage members to feel different textures, then demonstrate how to imitate the foods.

VOICE	LARYNGECTOMY	**PHYSICAL DISABILITY**	**PHONOLOGICAL IMPAIRMENT**	MENTAL ILLNESS	**HEARING IMPAIRMENT**
STUTTER	DYSPHASIA	**LEARNING DISABILITY**	DYSPRAXIA DYSARTHRIA	ELDERLY	**LANGUAGE IMPAIRMENT**

Foundation Skills
gelling
eye-contact
posture
facial expression
gesture
space/proximity
listening (basic)
volume, prosody, tone, pitch
memory

Interaction Skills
greetings
initiation/asking questions
listening/reflecting back, responding
answering questions/responding
termination
co-operating
turn-taking

Affective Skills
disclosures

Cognitive Skills

11. FINDING OUT

Members of the group are divided into pairs and each member is instructed to find out three things that they didn't already know about their partner. This information is to be obtained by asking each other questions. Members of the group are to remember the three things and not write them down. They are allowed 5 minutes to complete the task. The group then re-forms and each member introduces his partner to the rest of the group and relates the three pieces of information.

Modifications
To simplify:
• Specify the information which the members are to find out, e.g. name of partner, favourite food, place of birth.
• Reduce the number of things the members are to find out, e.g. find out one thing about your partner.
• Combine the above two, i.e. ask for *one* specific piece of information, e.g. favourite food.
• Therapist and a helper model questions that the group members might ask each other.

Non-verbal clients:
• Use alternative communication systems, e.g. charts or signing to encourage non-verbal members to question each other. Helpers may be required to assist.

VOICE	LARYNGECTOMY	PHYSICAL DISABILITY	PHONOLOGICAL IMPAIRMENT	MENTAL ILLNESS	HEARING IMPAIRMENT
STUTTER	DYSPHASIA	LEARNING DISABILITY	DYSPRAXIA DYSARTHRIA	ELDERLY	LANGUAGE IMPAIRMENT

Foundation Skills	Interaction Skills
observation	
eye-contact	
posture	
presentation	
facial expression	
gesture	
touch	
memory	

Affective Skills	Cognitive Skills
	problem solving

12. IN THE MANNER OF THE WORD

One person leaves the room. The rest of the group sits in a circle and decides on an adverb, e.g. unhappily, slowly. The person is invited back into the room and asks individual group members to perform various actions 'in the manner of the word', e.g. 'Joe, comb your hair in the manner of the word' and Joe combs his hair unhappily or slowly. The person has to guess what the adverb is.

Modifications
To simplify:
• The therapist suggests three simple adverbs, e.g. quickly, slowly, happily. One member leaves the room and the group chooses one of the three suggested adverbs. When the group member returns to the room, he then has to consider only one of three choices.
• The therapist gives the person outside the room suggestions for actions, e.g. brushing teeth, making a telephone call, etc.

Limited verbal comprehension:
• The therapist and helper demonstrate the exercise.

VOICE	LARYNGECTOMY	PHYSICAL DISABILITY	PHONOLOGICAL IMPAIRMENT	MENTAL ILLNESS	HEARING IMPAIRMENT
STUTTER	DYSPHASIA	LEARNING DISABILITY	DYSPRAXIA DYSARTHRIA	ELDERLY	LANGUAGE IMPAIRMENT

Foundation Skills	Interaction Skills
observation	
posture	
presentation	
relaxation	
memory	

Affective Skills	Cognitive Skills

13. WALK IN THE SAME STYLE

The group stands in a large circle and one member is instructed to walk around the inside of the circle whilst the others observe. The rest of the group then attempts to walk in the style of that person. This is repeated a few times and then the group reassembles to discuss posture.

Modifications
To simplify:
Limited verbal comprehension:
• The therapist demonstrates, imitating one member.

Limited mobility:
• The group observes and then imitates a standing or a seated posture.

VOICE	LARYNGECTOMY	**PHYSICAL** **DISABILITY**	PHONOLOGICAL IMPAIRMENT	**MENTAL** **ILLNESS**	**HEARING** **IMPAIRMENT**
STUTTER	**DYSPHASIA**	**LEARNING** **DISABILITY**	DYSPRAXIA DYSARTHRIA	**ELDERLY**	**LANGUAGE** **IMPAIRMENT**

Foundation Skills
gelling
observation
eye-contact
posture
facial expression
gesture
listening
volume, prosody, tone, pitch
memory

Interaction Skills
initiation
topic maintenance/repair of
    conversations
termination
co-operating
turn-taking

Affective Skills

Cognitive Skills
social perception

14. BUILD A STORY

The group is seated in a circle. A story is to be created by each member saying one sentence in turn, with an appropriate accompanying gesture or mime, e.g. (1)'One day I woke up' (stretch arms out and yawn). (2)'I went downstairs to make a cup of tea' (stamp feet, mime pouring out tea). The story continues with each member adding a sentence and the last member should give an appropriate concluding sentence.

Modification
To simplify:
• Use picture sequencing cards to aid sentence construction.

VOICE	LARYNGECTOMY	PHYSICAL DISABILITY	PHONOLOGICAL IMPAIRMENT	MENTAL ILLNESS	HEARING IMPAIRMENT
STUTTER	DYSPHASIA	LEARNING DISABILITY	DYSPRAXIA DYSARTHRIA	ELDERLY	LANGUAGE IMPAIRMENT

Foundation Skills
observation
eye-contact
posture
facial expression
gesture
space/proximity
listening
volume, prosody, tone, pitch
touch

Interaction Skills
initiation/asking questions
listening/reflecting back, responding
answering questions/responding
topic maintenance/repair of
    conversations
termination
co-operating
turn-taking, breaking in, interrupting

Affective Skills
identification of feelings
recognizing own feelings
recognizing feelings of others
disclosures

Cognitive Skills
social peception
problem solving
self-instruction
assertion

15. LET ME IN

The group is divided into subgroups of three who should be seated in
the following way:

```
            ┌───┐
            │ 3 │
            └───┘

      ┌───┐     ┌───┐
      │ 1 │     │ 2 │
      └───┘     └───┘
```

Members number 1 and 2 are instructed to hold a conversation with
each other and not allow number 3 to break in. Number 3 is instructed
to make every effort to interrupt the conversation. After two minutes, the
group reforms to discuss their feelings in the different roles. This activity
provides a starting point for a discussion of turn-taking.

Modification
• Various roles may be allocated to each member, e.g. mother, father
  and child.

VOICE	LARYNGECTOMY	PHYSICAL DISABILITY	PHONOLOGICAL IMPAIRMENT	MENTAL ILLNESS	HEARING IMPAIRMENT
STUTTER	DYSPHASIA	LEARNING DISABILITY	DYSPRAXIA DYSARTHRIA	ELDERLY	LANGUAGE IMPAIRMENT

Foundation Skills	Interaction Skills
observation	asking questions
eye-contact	listening, responding
presentation/grooming	answering questions/responding
gesture	co-operating
listening	turn-taking
memory	

Affective Skills	Cognitive Skills
	social perception
	problem solving
	self-instruction

16. HOW MANY?

The group is seated in a circle and the leader will ask each member in turn a question relating to the group member, e.g., 'How many people have brown hair?', 'How many people are wearing trousers?'. The member being questioned will need to observe the group in order to give a correct response. The question-master may be changed and the exercise repeated.

VOICE	LARYNGECTOMY	PHYSICAL DISABILITY	PHONOLOGICAL IMPAIRMENT	MENTAL ILLNESS	HEARING IMPAIRMENT
STUTTER	DYSPHASIA	LEARNING DISABILITY	DYSPRAXIA DYSARTHRIA	ELDERLY	LANGUAGE IMPAIRMENT

Foundation Skills
gelling
observation
eye-contact
posture
facial expression
gesture
space/proximity
listening
volume, prosody, tone, pitch
touch
memory

Interaction Skills
initiation
topic maintenance
termination
co-operating
turn-taking

Affective Skills
identification of feelings
recognizing feelings of others
trust

Cognitive Skills
social perception
problem solving
self-instruction
self-monitoring evaluation and
    reinforcement

17. ANOTHER PAIR OF HANDS

The group is divided into pairs and seated in a semi-circle. The first pair stand before the group, one in front of the other. The person standing in front is instructed to hold his hands behind his back and talk on any topic for 30 seconds. At the same time his partner will place his arms around him and will provide appropriate gestures for what is being said. When each pair has had a turn, the group reforms to discuss the use of gesture. To extend the exercise, roles can be reversed within each pair.

Modification
To simplify:
• Simple statements should be used, e.g. I am yawning, I am cold.

VOICE	LARYNGECTOMY	**PHYSICAL DISABILITY**	**PHONOLOGICAL IMPAIRMENT**	**MENTAL ILLNESS**	**HEARING IMPAIRMENT**
STUTTER	DYSPHASIA	**LEARNING DISABILITY**	**DYSPRAXIA** DYSARTHRIA	ELDERLY	**LANGUAGE IMPAIRMENT**

Foundation Skills	**Interaction Skills**
facial expression	co-operating
gesture	turn-taking
listening	
volume, prosody, tone, pitch	
memory	

Affective Skills	**Cognitive Skills**
identification of feelings	social perception
recognizing own feelings	self-instruction
trust	self-monitoring evaluation and
disclosures	reinforcement
	assertion

18. MODE OF TRANSPORT

Group members are asked to consider various modes and types of transport, e.g. car, aeroplane, train, etc., and to choose the one that most accurately reflects how they are feeling at that particular moment. They should also consider what the vehicle looks like and where it is, e.g. 'I am a red Volkswagon beetle car in a traffic jam in London'. These can be written down or remembered. Each member in turn then describes his vehicle to the group and a discussion regarding identification of feelings should follow.

Modification

To simplify:

• Group members may choose their mode of transport from a selection of pictures.

VOICE	LARYNGECTOMY	PHYSICAL DISABILITY	PHONOLOGICAL IMPAIRMENT	MENTAL ILLNESS	HEARING IMPAIRMENT
STUTTER	DYSPHASIA	LEARNING DISABILITY	DYSPRAXIA DYSARTHRIA	ELDERLY	LANGUAGE IMPAIRMENT

Foundation Skills
observation
eye-contact
posture
facial expression
gesture

Interaction Skills
co-operating
turn-taking

Affective Skills
identification of feelings
recognizing own feelings
recognizing feelings of others

Cognitive Skills
social perception
problem solving

19. GUESS THE MIME

The group is seated in a semicircle and a topic is chosen, e.g. thing we
don't like doing. Each member will stand in front of the group in turn
and mime his dislike, e.g. 'Washing my hair'. The rest of the group have
to guess the mime.

Modification
To simplify:
• Pictures may be used to help group members with their mime.

VOICE	LARYNGECTOMY	**PHYSICAL DISABILITY**	**PHONOLOGICAL IMPAIRMENT**	**MENTAL ILLNESS**	**HEARING IMPAIRMENT**
STUTTER	DYSPHASIA	**LEARNING DISABILITY**	**DYSPRAXIA** DYSARTHRIA	ELDERLY	**LANGUAGE IMPAIRMENT**

Foundation Skills
gelling
observation
eye-contact
posture
facial expression
gesture
space/proximity
listening
volume, prosody, tone, pitch
memory

Interaction Skills
initiation/asking questions
listening/reflecting back, responding
answering questions/responding
topic maintenance/repair of
     conversations
termination
turn-taking, breaking in, interrupting
co-operating

Affective Skills
identification of feelings
recognizing own feelings
recognizing feelings of others

Cognitive Skills
social perception
self-instruction
self-monitoring evaluation and
     reinforcement
assertion

20. EYE GAZE

The group is divided into pairs and partners are to talk to each other for
three minutes. For the first minute, they are instructed not to look at
each other; for the second minute, they are to maintain continuous eye
gaze and for the third minute, they should use normal eye contact. The
leader will signal at each minute interval. The group re-forms to discuss
appropriate eye contact.

Modification
To simplify:
• Members should be instructed to say one sentence to each other.

VOICE	LARYNGECTOMY	PHYSICAL DISABILITY	PHONOLOGICAL IMPAIRMENT	MENTAL ILLNESS	HEARING IMPAIRMENT
STUTTER	DYSPHASIA	LEARNING DISABILITY	DYSPRAXIA DYSARTHRIA	ELDERLY	LANGUAGE IMPAIRMENT

Foundation Skills   **Interaction Skills**
observation
posture
facial expression
gesture
space/proximity
listening

Affective Skills   **Cognitive Skills**
identification of feelings   social perception

21. WHERE DO WE STAND?

A selection of large pictures should be prepared, e.g. pictures of famous people, different types of food, places to visit, types of transport, etc. One picture is placed in the centre of the room. A member of the group is asked to position himself in the room and adopt a posture and facial expression that demonstrates how he feels about that picture, i.e. stand far away from a picture of jelly with a look of disgust (indicating the person dislikes jelly). The remaining group members should then describe what the posture and position discloses about that person's feelings.

VOICE	LARYNGECTOMY	PHYSICAL DISABILITY	PHONOLOGICAL IMPAIRMENT	MENTAL ILLNESS	HEARING IMPAIRMENT
STUTTER	DYSPHASIA	LEARNING DISABILITY	DYSPRAXIA DYSARTHRIA	ELDERLY	LANGUAGE IMPAIRMENT

Foundation Skills
gelling
observation
posture
space/proximity
listening
touch
memory

Interaction Skills
co-operating

Affective Skills

Cognitive Skills
problem solving
negotiating

22. NUMBERS ON THE FLOOR

The group stands in a circle with the leader standing in the centre. The leader calls out a number and all members in the circle should place that number of parts of their body on the floor, e.g. call 4: members place their hands on the floor making 4 contacts (2 hands and 2 feet). This can also be carried out in small groups of 2 to 4 requiring co-operation and negotiation between groups.

VOICE	LARYNGECTOMY	PHYSICAL DISABILITY	**PHONOLOGICAL IMPAIRMENT**	MENTAL ILLNESS	**HEARING IMPAIRMENT**
STUTTER	DYSPHASIA	**LEARNING DISABILITY**	**DYSPRAXIA** DYSARTHRIA	ELDERLY	**LANGUAGE IMPAIRMENT**

Foundation Skills
gelling
observation
eye-contact
gesture
space/proximity
listening
volume, prosody, tone, pitch
memory

Interaction Skills
asking questions
listening, responding
co-operating
turn-taking

Affective Skills

Cognitive Skills
problem solving
self-instruction
self-monitoring evaluation and
reinforcement
negotiating

23. DRAW A HOUSE

The group is divided into pairs and one member instructs his partner on how to draw a house. The person who is drawing should only carry out instructions given by his partner. When the task is completed roles should be reversed. The group then re-forms to discuss the giving and receiving of verbal instructions.

Modification
To simplify:
• Instructions to draw a shape, e.g. square, triangle.

VOICE	LARYNGECTOMY	PHYSICAL DISABILITY	PHONOLOGICAL IMPAIRMENT	MENTAL ILLNESS	HEARING IMPAIRMENT
STUTTER	DYSPHASIA	LEARNING DISABILITY	DYSPRAXIA DYSARTHRIA	ELDERLY	LANGUAGE IMPAIRMENT

Foundation Skills	Interaction Skills
gelling	greetings
observation	co-operating
eye-contact	turn-taking
posture	
presentation/grooming	
facial expression	
gesture	
space/proximity	
listening	
volume, prosody, tone, pitch	
touch	
memory	

Affective Skills	Cognitive Skills
	assertion

24. GREETINGS

The group is instructed to move around the room. At a signal from the leader they should stop and introduce themselves to a fellow group member, e.g. 'Hello, my name is Elaine'. The exercise continues until all members have introduced themselves to each other.

VOICE	LARYNGECTOMY	PHYSICAL DISABILITY	PHONOLOGICAL IMPAIRMENT	MENTAL ILLNESS	HEARING IMPAIRMENT
STUTTER	DYSPHASIA	LEARNING DISABILITY	DYSPRAXIA DYSARTHRIA	ELDERLY	LANGUAGE IMPAIRMENT

Foundation Skills
gelling
observation
eye-contact
facial expression
gesture
listening
memory

Interaction Skills
greetings
co-operating
turn-taking

Affective Skills

Cognitive Skills
social perception

25. INTRODUCTIONS

The group is seated in a circle. The leader says her name, e.g. 'I'm Jane'. The next person says his name and then Jane's name, e.g. 'I'm John and this is Jane'. The next person says 'I'm George, this is John and that is Jane'. This continues until all members have given their name and the name of the other group members.

Modification
To simplify:
• Members each say their own name and that of the person preceding them.

VOICE	LARYNGECTOMY	PHYSICAL DISABILITY	PHONOLOGICAL IMPAIRMENT	MENTAL ILLNESS	HEARING IMPAIRMENT
STUTTER	DYSPHASIA	LEARNING DISABILITY	DYSPRAXIA DYSARTHRIA	ELDERLY	LANGUAGE IMPAIRMENT

Foundation Skills
gelling
observation
eye-contact
posture
facial expression
gesture
space/proximity
touch

Interaction Skills
co-operating
turn-taking

Affective Skills
identification of feelings
recognizing own feelings
recognizing feelings of others
disclosures

Cognitive Skills
social perception
problem solving
self-instruction
self-monitoring evaluation and
    reinforcement
assertion

26. WHO FEELS THE SAME?

Cards should be prepared with different emotions written on them, e.g.
happy, sad, bored, angry, tired. Each emotion is written on to two cards.
The pairs of cards are then shuffled and each group member is given one
card. The participants move round the room miming the emotion on
their card. The aim of the exercise is for each member to find the other
person who is miming the same emotion. When everyone has found
their partner, the group discusses non-verbal ways of expressing
emotions.

Modification
To simplify:
• Use paired pictures of emotions.

VOICE	LARYNGECTOMY	PHYSICAL DISABILITY	PHONOLOGICAL IMPAIRMENT	MENTAL ILLNESS	HEARING IMPAIRMENT
STUTTER	DYSPHASIA	LEARNING DISABILITY	DYSPRAXIA DYSARTHRIA	ELDERLY	LANGUAGE IMPAIRMENT

Foundation Skills	**Interaction Skills**
observation	listening, responding
eye-contact	co-operating
posture	turn-taking
facial expression	
gesture	
listening	
volume prosody, tone, pitch	

Affective Skills	**Cognitive Skills**
identification of feelings	social perception
recognizing feelings of others	self-instruction

27. GUESS WHAT!

Cards are prepared with written statements. The statements should be varied with both good and bad incidents, e.g.:

* 'I have won a hundred pounds'.
* I am going on a world cruise'.
* My cat is ill'.
* My car has broken down'.

Each group member is given a card and one person is selected to read out the statement on his card. Each remaining group member is asked to make an appropriate response to the statement, e.g. 'How wonderful!', 'You lucky thing!', 'You must be worried!', 'How awful!'. When all members have read their statements and the group has responded, a full discussion should take place on how to respond appropriately to others' good or bad news.

VOICE	LARYNGECTOMY	PHYSICAL DISABILITY	PHONOLOGICAL IMPAIRMENT	MENTAL ILLNESS	HEARING IMPAIRMENT
STUTTER	DYSPHASIA	LEARNING DISABILITY	DYSPRAXIA DYSARTHRIA	ELDERLY	LANGUAGE IMPAIRMENT

Foundation Skills
gelling
eye-contact
posture
space/proximity
touch

Interaction Skills
co-operating
breaking in, interrupting

Affective Skills
identification of feelings
recognizing own feelings
recognizing feelings of others
trust
disclosures

Cognitive Skills
problem solving
assertion

28. BREAKING INTO THE CIRCLE

A volunteer is instructed to stand outside the group. The rest of the group stand in a circle, link arms and close any gaps between them. The 'outsider' is to try to break into the circle whilst the rest of the group are to prevent him from doing so. After a short time, the 'outsider' is asked to describe his feelings. The group reforms into a linked circle including the 'outsider'. The difficulties experienced by people with communication problems, which would include isolation and exclusion from group interaction, are then discussed.

VOICE	LARYNGECTOMY	PHYSICAL DISABILITY	PHONOLOGICAL IMPAIRMENT	MENTAL ILLNESS	HEARING IMPAIRMENT
STUTTER	DYSPHASIA	LEARNING DISABILITY	DYSPRAXIA DYSARTHRIA	ELDERLY	LANGUAGE IMPAIRMENT

Foundation Skills
gelling
observation
eye-contact
facial expression
gesture
space/proximity
listening
volume, prosody, tone, pitch
relaxation
touch
memory

Interaction Skills
initiation/asking questions
listening/reflecting back, responding
answering questions/responding
topic maintenance
termination
complimenting
co-operating
turn-taking

Affective Skills
identification of feelings
recognizing own feelings
recognizing feelings of others
trust
disclosures

Cognitive Skills
social perception
self-monitoring, evaluation and
  reinforcement
assertion

29. THE PRAISE GAME

The group divides into pairs and the members are instructed that they are to converse with their partner for five minutes. During the conversation they should praise or make a positive statement to each other. The group then re-forms and each person is asked what praise they received and their partner is asked how they reacted. The group then discusses giving and receiving praise.

VOICE	LARYNGECTOMY	PHYSICAL DISABILITY	PHONOLOGICAL IMPAIRMENT	MENTAL ILLNESS	HEARING IMPAIRMENT
STUTTER	DYSPHASIA	LEARNING DISABILITY	DYSPRAXIA DYSARTHRIA	ELDERLY	LANGUAGE IMPAIRMENT

Foundation Skills	Interaction Skills
observation	co-operation
eye-contact	turn-taking
posture	
presentation	
facial expression	
gesture	
space/proximity	
touch	

Affective Skills	Cognitive Skills
identification of feelings	social perception
recognizing own feelings	problem solving
recognizing feelings of others	
trust	

30. PUPPETS

Cards are prepared with various emotions written on them, e.g. happy, angry, afraid, excited, sad. The group is divided into pairs and seated in a circle with each member next to his partner. Each pair is given a card and instructed that one person is to be a 'puppet' whilst the partner will position and arrange him in such a way in order to demonstrate the emotion on the card. This will include posture and facial expression. The remainder of the group is to guess the emotion. When all pairs have completed the task, the group discusses how emotions are shown non-verbally.

Modification
Non-readers:
• Use pictures rather than the written word.

VOICE	LARYNGECTOMY	PHYSICAL DISABILITY	**PHONOLOGICAL IMPAIRMENT**	MENTAL ILLNESS	**HEARING IMPAIRMENT**
STUTTER	DYSPHASIA	**LEARNING DISABILITY**	**DYSPRAXIA** DYSARTHRIA	ELDERLY	**LANGUAGE IMPAIRMENT**

Foundation Skills   **Interaction Skills**
observation   co-operating
eye-contact
posture
facial expression
gesture

Affective Skills   **Cognitive Skills**
                               problem solving

31. WHO STARTED IT?

One group member is asked to leave the room while the rest of the
group is instructed to choose a leader. The leader will be required to
start an action, e.g. clapping, foot stamping, which the rest of the group
will copy. The leader must change the action periodically and the rest of
the group should follow suit. The person outside the room will be asked
to return and guess which person is the leader, initiating the actions.
When the correct leader has been identified, the exercise is repeated
with different members taking over the two individual roles.

VOICE	LARYNGECTOMY	PHYSICAL DISABILITY	PHONOLOGICAL IMPAIRMENT	MENTAL ILLNESS	HEARING IMPAIRMENT
STUTTER	DYSPHASIA	LEARNING DISABILITY	DYSPRAXIA DYSARTHRIA	ELDERLY	

Foundation Skills
observation
facial expression
gesture
listening
volume, prosody, tone, pitch

Interaction Skills
co-operating
turn-taking

Affective Skills
identification of feelings
recognizing own feelings
recognizing feelings of others

Cognitive Skills
self-instruction
self-monitoring

32. LIKES AND DISLIKES

The group is seated in a circle and each member is instructed to take a turn in saying one positive thing and one negative thing about food, school, work or television, e.g. 'I *love* peanuts but I *hate* olives'. Each person exaggerates the word 'love' and 'hate', using appropriate facial expression and tone of voice. The group then discusses how feelings are expressed, both verbally and non-verbally.

Modification
To simplify:
• Each group member says the same sentence using appropriate non-verbal skills.

VOICE	LARYNGECTOMY	PHYSICAL DISABILITY	PHONOLOGICAL IMPAIRMENT	MENTAL ILLNESS	HEARING IMPAIRMENT
STUTTER	DYSPHASIA	LEARNING DISABILITY	DYSPRAXIA DYSARTHRIA	ELDERLY	LANGUAGE IMPAIRMENT

Foundation Skills
gelling
observation
eye-contact
posture
facial expression
gesture
space/proximity
listening
volume, prosody, tone, pitch

Interaction Skills
greetings
co-operating
turn-taking

Affective Skills

Cognitive Skills
social perception

33. SPEAK UP!

The group is divided into pairs. One partner is required to say, 'Hello, my name is . . ., what is yours?' several times, varying their volume. The first time they should say it very quietly, then repeat it, increasing the volume each time until they are shouting. The other person is required to listen and respond non-verbally according to whether it is too quiet, appropriate or too loud. Partners then change roles. The group then reforms and discusses appropriate volume and cues from listeners which are helpful in modifying volume.

VOICE	LARYNGECTOMY	PHYSICAL DISABILITY	PHONOLOGICAL IMPAIRMENT	MENTAL ILLNESS	HEARING IMPAIRMENT
STUTTER	DYSPHASIA	LEARNING DISABILITY	DYSPRAXIA DYSARTHRIA	ELDERLY	LANGUAGE IMPAIRMENT

Foundation Skills	Interaction Skills
gelling	co-operating
observation	turn-taking
eye-contact	
facial expression	
gesture	
space/proximity	
memory	

Affective Skills	Cognitive Skills

34. PASS THE GESTURE

The group is seated in a circle. One member makes a simple body movement or gesture, e.g. clap, nod. The person seated to the right makes the same gesture and then makes his own gesture. This continues around the circle until the last person has to perform the actions of each member of the group in sequence.

Modifications
To simplify:
• Divide into smaller groups so fewer actions will need to be remembered.

Limited mobility:
• Use facial expressions or actions involving functional body parts.

VOICE	LARYNGECTOMY	**PHYSICAL DISABILITY**	**PHONOLOGICAL IMPAIRMENT**	MENTAL ILLNESS	**HEARING IMPAIRMENT**
STUTTER	DYSPHASIA	**LEARNING DISABILITY**	**DYSPRAXIA** DYSARTHRIA	ELDERLY	**LANGUAGE IMPAIRMENT**

Foundation Skills
observation
eye-contact
facial expression
space/proximity

Interaction Skills
co-operating

Affective Skills
identification of feelings
recognizing own feelings
recognizing feelings of others

Cognitive Skills
social perception

35. ADVANCING

The group stands in two lines on either side of the room facing one another. They are then instructed to advance towards one another and stop when they feel they are at a comfortable distance from their partner. Variations in distance between the pairs are then observed and the group discusses appropriate and inappropriate proximity.

VOICE	LARYNGECTOMY	PHYSICAL DISABILITY	PHONOLOGICAL IMPAIRMENT	MENTAL ILLNESS	HEARING IMPAIRMENT
STUTTER	DYSPHASIA	LEARNING DISABILITY	DYSPRAXIA DYSARTHRIA	ELDERLY	LANGUAGE IMPAIRMENT

Foundation Skills
observation
eye-contact
posture
facial expression
gesture
space/proximity
listening
volume, tone
relaxation
touch

Interaction Skills
co-operating

Affective Skills
recognizing feelings of others
trust

Cognitive Skills
problem solving
reinforcement

36. FREEZE!

The group is divided into pairs and sit opposite one another. One person from each pair is then instructed to 'freeze', i.e., remain rigidly in a posture for 10 seconds. Their partner is then instructed to help them adopt a comfortable relaxed posture, giving verbal instructions and physical prompts. The group then discusses posture and relaxation.

VOICE	LARYNGECTOMY	PHYSICAL DISABILITY	PHONOLOGICAL IMPAIRMENT	MENTAL ILLNESS	HEARING IMPAIRMENT
STUTTER	DYSPHASIA	LEARNING DISABILITY	DYSPRAXIA DYSARTHRIA	ELDERLY	LANGUAGE IMPAIRMENT

Foundation Skills
observation
eye-contact
facial expression
gesture
space/proximity
listening
volume, prosody, tone, pitch
memory

Interaction Skills
initiation/asking questions
listening/reflecting back, responding
answering questions/responding
topic maintenance/repair of
    conversations
termination
co-operating
turn-taking, breaking in, interrupting

Affective Skills

Cognitive Skills
social perception

37. THE MICROPHONE

The group is arranged in a circle and a seating plan is drawn on a blackboard. The members are required to discuss a topic, e.g. a television programme, holidays, but they can only speak if they are holding the microphone which can be represented by a ruler. The microphone must therefore be handed around to those who wish to say something. The group leader charts the progress of the microphone around the group on the blackboard. On completion of the topic, the group is able to see from the diagram how the various members participated. A discussion on turn-taking should then follow.

Modification
Limited mobility:
• Members signal when they wish to speak and a helper moves around the group with the microphone.

VOICE	LARYNGECTOMY	**PHYSICAL DISABILITY**	**PHONOLOGICAL IMPAIRMENT**	**MENTAL ILLNESS**	**HEARING IMPAIRMENT**
STUTTER	**DYSPHASIA**	**LEARNING DISABILITY**	**DYSPRAXIA DYSARTHRIA**	**ELDERLY**	**LANGUAGE IMPAIRMENT**

Foundation Skills
observation
eye-contact
facial expression
listening
volume, prosody, tone, pitch
memory
gesture

Interaction Skills
initiation/asking questions
listening/reflecting back, responding
answering questions/responding
co-operating
turn-taking

Affective Skills

Cognitive Skills
problem solving

38. WHAT IS MY JOB?

The group is seated in a circle and one member leaves the room. The remaining participants choose a job for that person and then invite him back. Each member of the group then asks the person a question as if they were interviewing them for the agreed job, without telling him what that job is, e.g. if the job chosen is a fireman, the questions could be:

- 'Do you enjoy climbing?'
- 'Do you like wearing a uniform?'
- 'Do you enjoy fast driving?'

The interviewee tries to guess what the job is before another member has a turn.

VOICE	LARYNGECTOMY	PHYSICAL DISABILITY	PHONOLOGICAL IMPAIRMENT	MENTAL ILLNESS	HEARING IMPAIRMENT
STUTTER	DYSPHASIA	LEARNING DISABILITY	DYSPRAXIA DYSARTHRIA	ELDERLY	LANGUAGE IMPAIRMENT

Foundation Skills
observation
posture
space/proximity
relaxation

Interaction Skills

Affective Skills

Cognitive Skills

39. CANDLES

Members of the group stand with adequate space around them. The leader then instructs them to imagine that they are a candle that is alight and slowly melting. As they melt, each person sinks to the floor.

Modification

To simplify:

* The therapist lights a real candle (e.g. birthday candle) and the group watches it melt. The group is then instructed to imitate this.

VOICE	LARYNGECTOMY	PHYSICAL DISABILITY	**PHONOLOGICAL IMPAIRMENT**	MENTAL ILLNESS	**HEARING IMPAIRMENT**
STUTTER	DYSPHASIA	**LEARNING DISABILITY**	**DYSPRAXIA** DYSARTHRIA	ELDERLY	**LANGUAGE IMPAIRMENT**

Foundation Skills   **Interaction Skills**
observation
posture
facial expression
gesture
space/proximity
listening

Affective Skills   **Cognitive Skills**
identification of feelings   social perception

40. HOW DO WE LOOK?

The group is seated in a circle. The leader describes a situation, e.g. listening to music; cheering a football team on television; waiting to be interviewed. Members are instructed to adopt a posture appropriate to each situation. The group then discusses variations of posture including use of facial expression and gesture.

Modification
To simplify:
• Therapist shows the group pictures of people sitting in various postures. The group imitate the posture and discuss appropriate posture for a given situation.

VOICE	LARYNGECTOMY	PHYSICAL DISABILITY	PHONOLOGICAL IMPAIRMENT	MENTAL ILLNESS	HEARING IMPAIRMENT
STUTTER	DYSPHASIA	LEARNING DISABILITY	DYSPRAXIA DYSARTHRIA	ELDERLY	LANGUAGE IMPAIRMENT

Foundation Skills
observation
eye-contact
posture
facial expression
gesture
space/proximity
touch

Interaction Skills
co-operating

Affective Skills
identification of feelings
recognizing feelings of others

Cognitive Skills
social perception
problem solving

41. HOW CLOSE SHOULD WE GET?

Cards are prepared describing scenarios relating to proximity in communication, e.g. comforting someone who is sad, talking to a stranger in a
shop, talking to a close friend, speaking to someone in high authority.
The group is seated in a circle and two members are given a card and
instructed to position themselves in the appropriate way. The remainder
of the group guess what is happening. A discussion should take place
after each presentation regarding proximity and factors which affect how
we position ourselves.

VOICE	LARYNGECTOMY	PHYSICAL DISABILITY	PHONOLOGICAL IMPAIRMENT	MENTAL ILLNESS	HEARING IMPAIRMENT
STUTTER	DYSPHASIA	LEARNING DISABILITY	DYSPRAXIA DYSARTHRIA	ELDERLY	LANGUAGE IMPAIRMENT

Foundation Skills   **Interaction Skills**
gelling   co-operating
observation
posture
space/proximity
touch

Affective Skills   **Cognitive Skills**
                               problem solving

42. TANGLE

Two members of the group leave the room. The other members of the group stand in a circle and join hands. The group are instructed to get into a tangle by going over and under the arches formed by the joined arms, without breaking contact. When the circle is sufficiently tangled, the two members are invited back into the room and instructed to untangle the people using verbal and physical means, without breaking the link.

VOICE	LARYNGECTOMY	PHYSICAL DISABILITY	**PHONOLOGICAL IMPAIRMENT**	MENTAL ILLNESS	**HEARING IMPAIRMENT**
STUTTER	DYSPHASIA	**LEARNING DISABILITY**	**DYSPRAXIA** DYSARTHRIA	ELDERLY	**LANGUAGE IMPAIRMENT**

Foundation Skills	Interaction Skills
gelling	co-operating
observation	
space/proximity	
touch	

Affective Skills	Cognitive Skills
trust	

43. THE GUIDING GAME

A simple obstacle course is set up, e.g. weaving around chairs. The group is split into pairs, one of whom will be the guide, the other, the 'blind' person. The 'blind' person is instructed to close his eyes while the guide manoeuvres him around the obstacle course, giving physical prompts but no verbal instructions. The partners then exchange roles.

Bmodification
To simplify:
* Instruct members to guide their partner across the room, avoiding one obstacle, e.g. a chair.

VOICE	LARYNGECTOMY	**PHYSICAL DISABILITY**	**PHONOLOGICAL IMPAIRMENT**	**MENTAL ILLNESS**	**HEARING IMPAIRMENT**
STUTTER	DYSPHASIA	**LEARNING DISABILITY**	**DYSPRAXIA** DYSARTHRIA	ELDERLY	**LANGUAGE IMPAIRMENT**

Foundation Skills	Interaction Skills
gelling	co-operating
observation	turn-taking
memory	

Affective Skills	Cognitive Skills

44. REMEMBER THE OBJECTS

A tray is prepared on which an assortment of objects (maximum eight) have been placed. The group sit in a circle and the tray is placed in the centre. The members have 30 seconds to observe what is on the tray. The tray is then removed; the group divides into pairs who are given 2 minutes to recall together which objects were on the tray. These may be written down. The group reassembles to discuss observation and memory.

Modifications

To simplify:
* Reduce the number of objects.
* Increase the time allowed for observation and recall.

VOICE	LARYNGECTOMY	**PHYSICAL DISABILITY**	PHONOLOGICAL IMPAIRMENT	**MENTAL ILLNESS**	**HEARING IMPAIRMENT**
STUTTER	**DYSPHASIA**	**LEARNING DISABILITY**	DYSPRAXIA DYSARTHRIA	**ELDERLY**	**LANGUAGE IMPAIRMENT**

Foundation Skills	**Interaction Skills**
gelling	co-operating
observation	turn-taking
memory	
Affective Skills	**Cognitive Skills**

45. ADD THE OBJECTS

A tray is prepared on which six assorted objects have been placed. The group sit in a circle, the tray is placed in the centre and members are instructed that they have 30 seconds to remember what is on the tray. The tray is then removed and six new objects are added. The members are then allowed a further 30 seconds to observe the tray before it is finally removed. The group divides into pairs who are instructed to recall the six original objects that were placed on the tray.

Modification

To simplify:

• Increase the time allowed for observation and recall.
• Reduce the number of objects.

VOICE	LARYNGECTOMY	**PHYSICAL DISABILITY**	PHONOLOGICAL IMPAIRMENT	**MENTAL ILLNESS**	**HEARING IMPAIRMENT**
STUTTER	**DYSPHASIA**	**LEARNING DISABILITY**	DYSPRAXIA DYSARTHRIA	**ELDERLY**	**LANGUAGE IMPAIRMENT**

Foundation Skills
observation
eye-contact
posture
facial expression
gesture
space/proximity
listening
volume, prosody, tone, pitch
touch

Interaction Skills
co-operating
turn-taking

Affective Skills

Cognitive Skills

46. THE BLAH BLAH GAME

The group is divided into pairs and members are instructed to hold a conversation with their partner about a given topic without using recognizable words, e.g. 'blah blah'. They are to use intonation, stress and non-verbal cues appropriate to the topic.

Ideas for topics:

* 'I'm going on holiday next week'.
* 'My cat needs feeding'.
* 'I'm going to get a new bicycle'.
* 'Please could you lend me your car?'

The group then reforms and discusses intonation, stress, facial expression, gesture and posture.

VOICE	LARYNGECTOMY	PHYSICAL DISABILITY	PHONOLOGICAL IMPAIRMENT	MENTAL ILLNESS	HEARING IMPAIRMENT
STUTTER	DYSPHASIA	LEARNING DISABILITY	DYSPRAXIA DYSARTHRIA	ELDERLY	LANGUAGE IMPAIRMENT

Foundation Skills
observation
eye-contact
posture
facial expression
gesture
space/proximity
listening
volume, prosody, tone, pitch

Interaction Skills
topic maintenance/repair of
    conversations
turn-taking, breaking in, interrupting

Affective Skills

Cognitive Skills
self-instruction
assertion

47. INTERRUPTION

The group is divided into sub-groups of three. The first member of the triad is instructed to engage in a monologue for 30 seconds whilst the second member constantly interrupts. The third member is to observe how the first member reacts. All members take a turn in each role. The group then re-forms to discuss turn-taking and repair of conversations.

Modification
To simplify:
- The speaker is instructed to say only one sentence which the second member interrupts once.

VOICE	LARYNGECTOMY	PHYSICAL DISABILITY	PHONOLOGICAL IMPAIRMENT	MENTAL ILLNESS	HEARING IMPAIRMENT
STUTTER	**DYSPHASIA**	**LEARNING DISABILITY**	DYSPRAXIA DYSARTHRIA	**ELDERLY**	**LANGUAGE IMPAIRMENT**

Foundation Skills	Interaction Skills
gelling	co-operating
observation	
eye-contact	
space/proximity	
listening	
touch	
memory	

Affective Skills	Cognitive Skills

48. FRUIT SALAD

The group is seated on chairs in a circle and each member chooses the name of a fruit. One member stands in the centre of the circle and his chair is removed. The group leader or a nominated member of the group calls out two fruits and the members who selected those fruits change places with each other. During this change-over, the person standing in the centre attempts to reach one of the empty chairs first; whoever is left without a chair must stand in the centre. If 'fruit salad' is called, all members of the circle must change places, including the person standing in the centre.

Modifications
* The exercise may be repeated using alternative groupings, e.g. stations, football teams, etc.

To simplify:
* Reduce the size of the group.
* Do not have the extra person in the middle.

Limited mobility:
* Each member is given a picture of a fruit. When the two fruits are called, both members hold up their pictures.
* When 'fruit salad' is called, all members hold up their pictures.

VOICE	LARYNGECTOMY	PHYSICAL DISABILITY	PHONOLOGICAL IMPAIRMENT	MENTAL ILLNESS	HEARING IMPAIRMENT
STUTTER	DYSPHASIA	LEARNING DISABILITY	DYSPRAXIA DYSARTHRIA	ELDERLY	LANGUAGE IMPAIRMENT

Foundation Skills
gelling
observation
eye-contact
posture
facial expression
gesture
space/proximity
touch
memory

Interaction Skills
co-operating
turn-taking

Affective Skills   **Cognitive Skills**

49. CHINESE GESTURES

The group is seated in a circle and all members are instructed to close
their eyes, except one member who is to initiate a gesture, mime or
facial expression. The initiator taps the member seated on his right who
observes the gesture and then presents the same gesture to the person
on his right. Having presented the gesture, members can observe the
continuation of the exercise. The final member enacts the gesture which
is then compared to the orignal.

Modification
To simplify:
• The group leader initiates a simple gesture or action, e.g. covering
  face with hands.

Limited mobility
• Use only functional body parts.

VOICE	LARYNGECTOMY	**PHYSICAL DISABILITY**	**PHONOLOGICAL IMPAIRMENT**	MENTAL ILLNESS	**HEARING IMPAIRMENT**
STUTTER	DYSPHASIA	**LEARNING DISABILITY**	**DYSPRAXIA** DYSARTHRIA	ELDERLY	**LANGUAGE IMPAIRMENT**

Foundation Skills	**Interaction Skills**
listening	
volume, prosody, tone, pitch	

Affective Skills	**Cognitive Skills**
	problem solving

50. HOW DO I SOUND?

Sentences are written on cards which will be used to demonstrate appropriate changes in volume of speech, e.g.:

* 'Could everybody please stop talking and listen for a moment.'.
* 'Don't wake the baby.'
* 'Could you turn the radio down please'.
* 'Isn't this lecture boring'.

Group members are given a card and asked to read the sentence using the appropriate volume. A discussion then follows on variation of volume according to the content of a sentence and the context in which it may occur.

VOICE	LARYNGECTOMY	PHYSICAL DISABILITY	PHONOLOGICAL IMPAIRMENT	MENTAL ILLNESS	HEARING IMPAIRMENT
STUTTER	DYSPHASIA	LEARNING DISABILITY	DYSPRAXIA DYSARTHRIA	ELDERLY	LANGUAGE IMPAIRMENT

Foundation Skills	Interaction Skills
gelling	co-operating
observation	
posture	
space	
listening	
memory	

Affective Skills	Cognitive Skills

51. THE OLD FAMILY COACH

The group is seated in a circle with a leader in the centre. The leader gives each member the name of a character, e.g. father, mother, son, cousin and then makes up a story about 'the old family coach'. When one of the characters is mentioned, the appropriate member stands up, turns around and then sits down again. When the leader mentions 'the old family coach' all group members stand up and turn around in unison and then sit down.

Modification
Limited mobility:
• Distribute pictures of animals to group members. Tell a simple story mentioning animals. Members must hold up the appropriate picture when their animal is mentioned. When the word 'zoo' or 'farm' is mentioned, all members hold up their pictures.

VOICE	LARYNGECTOMY	**PHYSICAL DISABILITY**	**PHONOLOGICAL IMPAIRMENT**	**MENTAL ILLNESS**	**HEARING IMPAIRMENT**
STUTTER	DYSPHASIA	**LEARNING DISABILITY**	**DYSPRAXIA** DYSARTHRIA	**ELDERLY**	**LANGUAGE IMPAIRMENT**

Foundation Skills   **Interaction Skills**
observation   turn-taking
eye-contact
presentation/grooming
listening
memory

Affective Skills   **Cognitive Skills**
                              social perception
                              problem solving

---

52. I'M GOING TO A PARTY

The group is seated in a circle and are instructed that they are to say 'I am going to a party wearing a . . .'. The group leader will tell each member if they are permitted to go according to a rule; the rule being that the member must name an article of clothing worn by the person seated to his left. The leader initiates the game and all members take a turn until everybody has discovered the rule.

Modification
To simplify:
• The leader looks in an obvious way at the person seated to the left.

VOICE	LARYNGECTOMY	PHYSICAL DISABILITY	PHONOLOGICAL IMPAIRMENT	MENTAL ILLNESS	HEARING IMPAIRMENT
STUTTER	DYSPHASIA	LEARNING DISABILITY	DYSPRAXIA DYSARTHRIA	ELDERLY	LANGUAGE IMPAIRMENT

Foundation Skills   **Interaction Skills**
gelling   co-operating
observation   turn-taking
posture
gesture
space/proximity
listening
touch
memory

Affective Skills   **Cognitive Skills**
                                problem solving
                                negotiating

53. TEAM MACHINE

The group is divided into sub-groups of 3 – 5 members. Each sub-group is allowed 5 – 10 minutes to decide on a piece of equipment or machinery which they will corporately enact, e.g. typewriter, combine harvester; each member being a working part of the machine. Members are allowed to practise their choice of machine before demonstrating it to the main group, who are to guess what it is.

Modification
To simplify:
* Suggestions of machines and how to enact them are given.

VOICE	LARYNGECTOMY	**PHYSICAL DISABILITY**	**PHONOLOGICAL IMPAIRMENT**	MENTAL ILLNESS	**HEARING IMPAIRMENT**
STUTTER	DYSPHASIA	**LEARNING DISABILITY**	**DYSPRAXIA** DYSARTHRIA	ELDERLY	**LANGUAGE IMPAIRMENT**

Foundation Skills   **Interaction Skills**
gelling   co-operating
observation   turn-taking
eye-contact
posture
facial expression
space/proximity
listening
memory

Affective Skills   **Cognitive Skills**

54. THE NAME GAME

The group stands in a circle, each member wearing a label with their name clearly printed on it. The group leader commences the exercise by giving his own name, looking at another group member, saying that person's name and throwing an object, e.g. ball, beanbag, to him. This continues until all members have participated.

VOICE	LARYNGECTOMY	PHYSICAL DISABILITY	PHONOLOGICAL IMPAIRMENT	MENTAL ILLNESS	HEARING IMPAIRMENT
STUTTER	DYSPHASIA	LEARNING DISABILITY	DYSPRAXIA DYSARTHRIA	ELDERLY	LANGUAGE IMPAIRMENT

Foundation Skills
observation
posture
presentation
facial expression
gesture
space/proximity
touch

Interaction Skills
co-operating
turn-taking

Affective Skills

Cognitive Skills
social perception
problem solving

55. WHAT HAVE WE HERE?

One group member leaves the room while the rest of the group arrange themselves in a static scenario, e.g. two cars have collided. The member is then invited back into the room to guess what the scene depicts.

Modification
To simplify:
• Use pictures of scenarios to assist group members.

VOICE	LARYNGECTOMY	PHYSICAL DISABILITY	PHONOLOGICAL IMPAIRMENT	MENTAL ILLNESS	HEARING IMPAIRMENT
STUTTER	DYSPHASIA	LEARNING DISABILITY	DYSPRAXIA DYSARTHRIA	ELDERLY	LANGUAGE IMPAIRMENT

Foundation Skills	**Interaction Skills**
gelling	co-operating
space/proximity	turn-taking
listening	
memory	

Affective Skills	**Cognitive Skills**
identification of feelings	social perception
recognizing own feelings	self-monitoring evaluation and
recognizing feelings of others	reinforcement
trust	
disclosures	

56. GOOD POINTS

The group is divided into pairs and instructed to tell their partner three
good points about themselves, e.g. 'I have a sense of humour; I am good
at tennis; I am sympathetic'. Three minutes is allowed and the group
then re-forms and each member discloses his partner's three good
points to the main group.

Modification
To simplify:
• Reduce the number of good points to be disclosed.

VOICE	LARYNGECTOMY	PHYSICAL DISABILITY	PHONOLOGICAL IMPAIRMENT	MENTAL ILLNESS	HEARING IMPAIRMENT
STUTTER	DYSPHASIA	LEARNING DISABILITY	DYSPRAXIA DYSARTHRIA	ELDERLY	LANGUAGE IMPAIRMENT

Foundation Skills   **Interaction Skills**
gelling
observation
eye-contact
facial expression
listening

Affective Skills   **Cognitive Skills**

57. STOP AND STARE

The group is instructed to walk around the room and when the leader calls 'stop', the members are to establish eye-contact with the person nearest to them and maintain this whilst the leader counts aloud to three. They should then continue to walk around and the exercise is repeated.

VOICE	LARYNGECTOMY	PHYSICAL DISABILITY	PHONOLOGICAL IMPAIRMENT	MENTAL ILLNESS	HEARING IMPAIRMENT
STUTTER	DYSPHASIA	LEARNING DISABILITY	DYSPRAXIA DYSARTHRIA	ELDERLY	LANGUAGE IMPAIRMENT

Foundation Skills	**Interaction Skills**
listening	asking questions
memory	listening
	answering questions
	co-operating
	turn-taking

Affective Skills	**Cognitive Skills**
	problem solving

58. TWENTY QUESTIONS

The group sits in a circle and one member is invited to think of something, e.g., an object, person, animal, etc. They are then to state if it is an animal, vegetable or mineral and the rest of the group are instructed that they may ask no more than twenty questions to discover the answer. The questions can only have a 'yes' or 'no' response. One group member is allocated to count the number of questions. If a person thinks he knows the answer, he is allowed to guess, but if he is incorrect, it counts as a question. If nobody guesses after twenty questions, the person who thought of the object is the winner.

Modifications
To simplify:
• limit the category, e.g., suggest they think of a type of food or animal.

Limited verbal skills:
• discuss before the exercise how the questions should be formed, e.g., 'Is it a . . .?', 'Can it . . .?'.

VOICE	LARYNGECTOMY	**PHYSICAL DISABILITY**	PHONOLOGICAL IMPAIRMENT	**MENTAL ILLNESS**	**HEARING IMPAIRMENT**
STUTTER	DYSPHASIA	**LEARNING DISABILITY**	**DYSPRAXIA** DYSARTHRIA	**ELDERLY**	**LANGUAGE IMPAIRMENT**

Foundation Skills   **Interaction Skills**
facial expression   co-operating
gesture   turn-taking
listening
volume, prosody, tone, pitch
memory

Affective Skills   **Cognitive Skills**

59. WHAT DO WE MEAN?

The group is seated in a circle. A card with a sentence written on it is passed around and each member is asked to read the sentence changing the stress or intonation pattern, e.g.:

- *He* did not want to eat his dinner.
- He did not want to eat *his* dinner.
- He did not want to eat his *dinner*.
- He did not want to eat his dinner?

The group then discusses how intonation and stress affect the meaning of a sentence.

VOICE	LARYNGECTOMY	PHYSICAL DISABILITY	PHONOLOGICAL IMPAIRMENT	MENTAL ILLNESS	HEARING IMPAIRMENT
STUTTER	DYSPHASIA	LEARNING DISABILITY	DYSPRAXIA DYSARTHRIA	ELDERLY	LANGUAGE IMPAIRMENT

Foundation Skills	**Interaction Skills**
observation	co-operating
eye-contact	turn-taking
posture	
facial expression	
gesture	
space/proximity	
listening	
volume, prosody, tone, pitch	
memory	

Affective Skills	**Cognitive Skills**
	self-instruction
	self-monitoring evaluation and reinforcement

60. CHINESE TALES

The group are instructed that all but one member will be sent outside the room. The remaining person will listen to the group leader reading a sentence, e.g. 'It was a hot sunny day and the children were playing on the swings and the slide'. Another member is then called into the room and the first person will repeat what he heard the leader read out as accurately as possible. The third member is then called in and the second person then repeats the sentence to the third person. The exercise continues until each member has been called into the room. When every member has had a turn, the last person repeats what he has heard and the leader re-reads the original sentence. The group then discusses attention control, listening and memory skills.

Modification
To simplify:
• The leader should read out a short list of objects.

VOICE	LARYNGECTOMY	PHYSICAL DISABILITY	PHONOLOGICAL IMPAIRMENT	MENTAL ILLNESS	HEARING IMPAIRMENT
STUTTER	DYSPHASIA	LEARNING DISABILITY	DYSPRAXIA DYSARTHRIA	ELDERLY	LANGUAGE IMPAIRMENT

Foundation Skills
gelling
eye-contact
posture
facial expression
gesture
listening
volume, prosody, tone, pitch
memory

Interaction Skills
listening/reflecting back, responding
co-operating
turn-taking

Affective Skills
identification of feelings
recognizing own feelings
recognizing feelings of others

Cognitive Skills
social perception
problem solving
self-instruction

61. GOOD NEWS/BAD NEWS

The group is seated in a circle and is instructed that each member will take a turn to say some good news, and the person seated on their right will respond appropriately, with some bad news, e.g., 'The good news is that we have booked a holiday', 'The bad news is that I have lost the tickets'. Having said the bad news, the same person then continues with a statement of good news and the exercise proceeds until all group members have had a turn.

VOICE	LARYNGECTOMY	PHYSICAL DISABILITY	PHONOLOGICAL IMPAIRMENT	MENTAL ILLNESS	HEARING IMPAIRMENT
STUTTER	DYSPHASIA	LEARNING DISABILITY	DYSPRAXIA DYSARTHRIA	ELDERLY	LANGUAGE IMPAIRMENT

Foundation Skills
gelling
observation
eye-contact
posture
facial expression
gesture
listening
volume, prosody, tone, pitch
memory

Interaction Skills
initiation/asking questions
answering questions/responding
co-operating
turn-taking

Affective Skills
disclosures

Cognitive Skills
social perception
self-instruction
self-monitoring evaluation and
    reinforcement

62. QUESTIONS AND ANSWERS

The group is seated in a circle and members are instructed that the leader will ask the person seated on their right a question, e.g. 'What did you have for lunch?'. The question should be answered appropriately and that person then asks his neighbour the same question. The exercise continues until all group members have asked and responded to the same question.

Modification
To simplify:
• The question should be simplified, e.g. 'What is your name?', 'What is the time?'.

VOICE	LARYNGECTOMY	**PHYSICAL DISABILITY**	**PHONOLOGICAL IMPAIRMENT**	**MENTAL ILLNESS**	**HEARING IMPAIRMENT**
STUTTER	**DYSPHASIA**	**LEARNING DISABILITY**	**DYSPRAXIA DYSARTHRIA**	**ELDERLY**	**LANGUAGE IMPAIRMENT**

Foundation Skills
observation
eye-contact
facial expression
gesture
listening
volume, prosody, tone, pitch
memory

Interaction Skills
co-operating
turn-taking

Affective Skills
identification of feelings
recognizing own feelings
recognizing feelings of others
trust
disclosures

Cognitive Skills
social peception
self-instruction
self-monitoring evaluation and
    reinforcement
assertion

63. HOW DO YOU RATE?

The group is seated in a circle and is instructed that each member must rate how he is feeling at that time on a scale of one to 10. A rating of one denotes feeling low and 10 denotes feeling very good. Each member takes a turn giving his self-rating and disclosing the reasons for this. All the ratings may be added up and divided by the number of group members to give an average group rating of feelings. These group ratings may be compared during various sessions.

VOICE	LARYNGECTOMY	PHYSICAL DISABILITY	PHONOLOGICAL IMPAIRMENT	MENTAL ILLNESS	HEARING IMPAIRMENT
STUTTER	DYSPHASIA	LEARNING DISABILITY	DYSPRAXIA DYSARTHRIA	ELDERLY	LANGUAGE IMPAIRMENT

Foundation Skills
gelling
observation
eye-contact
space/proximity

Interaction Skills
co-operating
turn-taking

Affective Skills

Cognitive Skills

64. CHANGE PLACES

The group stands in a circle and one member is chosen to be the 'director'. The director winks at two members of the circle who should then change places with each other. Members need to observe the director closely to know when and with whom they should change places. After several turns, a different group member should become the director.

Modification
To simplify:
• The director points at the two members who are to change places.

VOICE	LARYNGECTOMY	PHYSICAL DISABILITY	PHONOLOGICAL IMPAIRMENT	MENTAL ILLNESS	HEARING IMPAIRMENT
STUTTER	DYSPHASIA	LEARNING DISABILITY	DYSPRAXIA DYSARTHRIA	ELDERLY	LANGUAGE IMPAIRMENT

Foundation Skills
gelling
observation
eye-contact
posture
facial expression
gesture
space/proximity
listening
volume, prosody, tone, pitch
touch
memory

Interaction Skills
co-operating
turn-taking

Affective Skills
identification of feelings
recognizing own feelings
recognizing feelings of others
trust

Cognitive Skills
social perception
self-instruction
assertion

65. MASTER AND SLAVE

The group is divided into pairs, one person being the master and one the slave. The master will instruct the slave to carry out tasks which the slave should obey, e.g. 'Sit on the floor', 'Stand on one leg'. However, if the slave does not wish to do the task or no longer wishes to continue being the slave, he can refuse and the roles then become reversed. The group re-forms to discuss feelings evoked in either the dominant or submissive role.

VOICE	LARYNGECTOMY	PHYSICAL DISABILITY	**PHONOLOGICAL IMPAIRMENT**	**MENTAL ILLNESS**	**HEARING IMPAIRMENT**
STUTTER	DYSPHASIA	**LEARNING DISABILITY**	**DYSPRAXIA** DYSARTHRIA	ELDERLY	**LANGUAGE IMPAIRMENT**

Foundation Skills   **Interaction Skills**
gelling   co-operating
observation   turn-taking
posture
space/proximity
touch
memory

Affective Skills   **Cognitive Skills**
identification of feelings   social perception
recognizing own feelings   self-instruction
recognizing feelings of others   assertion
trust

66. ROBOTS

The group is divided into pairs. One member of the pair is the master and his partner is the robot. The master will be in control of the robot's movements and signals to the robot which movement he must make. A tap on the right shoulder denotes walking to the right, a tap on the left shoulder denotes walking to the left and a tap on the centre of the robot's back denotes walking straight ahead. When the master touches the robot's head, this indicates that he is to stand still. The leader instructs the pair to move around the room and the master should ensure that the robot does not walk into another member of the group by controlling with appropriate taps. After two to three minutes, roles should be reversed. The group re-forms to discuss their feelings in the different roles.

VOICE	LARYNGECTOMY	PHYSICAL DISABILITY	**PHONOLOGICAL IMPAIRMENT**	**MENTAL ILLNESS**	**HEARING IMPAIRMENT**
STUTTER	DYSPHASIA	**LEARNING DISABILITY**	**DYSPRAXIA DYSARTHRIA**	ELDERLY	**LANGUAGE IMPAIRMENT**

Foundation Skills
observation
eye-contact
posture
presentation/grooming
facial expression
gesture
listening
volume, prosody, tone, pitch
memory

Interaction Skills
co-operating
turn-taking
complimenting

Affective Skills
identification of feelings
recognizing feelings of others
trust
disclosures

Cognitive Skills
social perception
assertion

67. THE PRAISE CIRCLE

The group is seated in a circle. The leader instructs the group that each member in turn is going to pay a compliment to the person sitting on his left and that person is to respond appropriately. The leader should start the exercise and when each member has had a turn the group should be encouraged to discuss how compliments can be thrown away or negated by a poor response from the recipient.

VOICE	LARYNGECTOMY	PHYSICAL DISABILITY	PHONOLOGICAL IMPAIRMENT	MENTAL ILLNESS	HEARING IMPAIRMENT
STUTTER	DYSPHASIA	LEARNING DISABILITY	DYSPRAXIA DYSARTHRIA	ELDERLY	LANGUAGE IMPAIRMENT

Foundation Skills
gelling
observation
eye-contact
posture
facial expression
gesture
space/proximity
listening (basic)
volume, prosody, tone, pitch
memory

Interaction Skills
initiation/asking questions
listening/reflecting back, responding
answering questions/responding
topic maintenance/repair of
    conversations
termination
complimenting
co-operating
turn-taking, breaking in, interrupting

Affective Skills
identification of feelings
recognizing own feelings
recognizing feelings of others
trust
disclosures

Cognitive Skills
social perception
problem solving
self-instruction
self-monitoring evaluation and
    reinforcement
negotiating
assertion

68. WHAT'S FOR SUPPER?

The group is divided into sub-groups of four people who are instructed that they have 5 minutes to negotiate what they will have for their evening meal. At the end of the allotted time, the groups reform and a spokesperson from each subgroup reports back the chosen meal and how the decision was reached. Group members should be given the opportunity to comment on their own level of participation in the discussion.

VOICE	LARYNGECTOMY	PHYSICAL DISABILITY	PHONOLOGICAL IMPAIRMENT	MENTAL ILLNESS	HEARING IMPAIRMENT
STUTTER	DYSPHASIA	LEARNING DISABILITY	DYSPRAXIA DYSARTHRIA	ELDERLY	LANGUAGE IMPAIRMENT

Foundation Skills
gelling
observation
eye-contact
posture
facial expression
gesture
space/proximity
listening (basic)
volume, prosody, tone, pitch
memory

Interaction Skills
initiation/asking questions
listening/reflecting back, responding
answering questions/responding
topic maintenance/repair of
    conversations
termination
complimenting
co-operating
turn-taking

Affective Skills
identification of feelings
recognizing own feelings
recognizing feelings of others
trust
disclosures

Cognitive Skills
social perception
problem solving
self-instruction
self-monitoring evaluation and
    reinforcement
negotiation
assertion

69. DESERT ISLAND

The group is seated in a circle and instructed that each member is allowed one minute to think of three individual items that they would wish to have if they were stranded on a desert island. This should not include people or animals. The group is then divided into pairs and each pair is to negotiate three items from the six they will have decided upon during the first part of the exercise. The group re-forms to discuss how decisions were made and whether the members felt they had been able to expression their views satisfactorily.

VOICE	LARYNGECTOMY	PHYSICAL DISABILITY	PHONOLOGICAL IMPAIRMENT	MENTAL ILLNESS	HEARING IMPAIRMENT
STUTTER	DYSPHASIA	LEARNING DISABILITY	DYSPRAXIA DYSARTHRIA	ELDERLY	LANGUAGE IMPAIRMENT

Foundation Skills
gelling
observation
eye-contact
posture
presentation/grooming
facial expression
gesture
space/proximity
memory

Interaction Skills
co-operating
turn-taking

Affective Skills

Cognitive Skills
social peception
problem solving

70. OBSERVATIONS

The group is divided into pairs and members are instructed to stand in two lines, each facing his partner. Line A members are instructed to hold a posture for half a minute whilst Line B members closely observe their partners. Line B are then instructed to turn their backs to their partner whilst Line A changes three aspects of their appearance:

- One to do with posture.
- One to do with clothing.
- One to do with facial expression.

Line B is then required to turn round and identify these changes. Roles are then reversed so that Line B holds the postures whilst Line A becomes the observers.

The group reconvenes to discuss feelings regarding both ability to observe easily and being observed.

Modification
To simplify:
- Instruct to change only one thing each time; suggest aspect to be changed, e.g. posture.

VOICE	LARYNGECTOMY	PHYSICAL DISABILITY	PHONOLOGICAL IMPAIRMENT	MENTAL ILLNESS	HEARING IMPAIRMENT
STUTTER	DYSPHASIA	LEARNING DISABILITY	DYSPRAXIA DYSARTHRIA	ELDERLY	LANGUAGE IMPAIRMENT

Foundation Skills	Interaction Skills
gelling	greetings
observation	initiation
eye-contact	co-operating
posture	turn-taking
facial expression	
gesture	
listening	
volume, prosody, tone, pitch	
memory	

Affective Skills	Cognitive Skills

71. PASS THE GREETING

The group is seated in a circle; the leader throws a ball to a member who should make a greeting statement, e.g. 'Hello, isn't it a nice day'. This person then throws the ball to another group member who will make a different greeting statement. The exercise continues until all members have had a turn. A discussion should follow on the use of greetings to initiate conversation.

Modification
Limited mobility:
• The leader should make eye-contact with the member who is to make the statement.

VOICE	LARYNGECTOMY	PHYSICAL DISABILITY	PHONOLOGICAL IMPAIRMENT	MENTAL ILLNESS	HEARING IMPAIRMENT
STUTTER	DYSPHASIA	LEARNING DISABILITY	DYSPRAXIA DYSARTHRIA	ELDERLY	LANGUAGE IMPAIRMENT

Foundation Skills
gelling
observation
eye-contact
posture
presentation/grooming
facial expression
gesture
space/proximity
listening
volume, prosody, tone, pitch
touch

Interaction Skills
initiation
listening/reflecting back, responding
answering questions/responding
complimenting
co-operating
turn-taking

Affective Skills
identification of feelings
recognizing own feelings
recognizing feelings of others
trust
disclosures

Cognitive Skills
social perception
self-instruction
self-monitoring evaluation and
    reinforcement
assertion

72. I CHOOSE YOU

Members of the group are instructed to find a partner and to make a
positive statement to their partner, e.g. 'I have chosen you because you
have a nice smile'. They should then approach another couple and each
member should make a positive statement to the new partners.

VOICE	LARYNGECTOMY	PHYSICAL DISABILITY	PHONOLOGICAL IMPAIRMENT	MENTAL ILLNESS	HEARING IMPAIRMENT
STUTTER	DYSPHASIA	LEARNING DISABILITY	DYSPRAXIA DYSARTHRIA	ELDERLY	LANGUAGE IMPAIRMENT

Foundation Skills
gelling
observation
eye-contact
posture
presentation/grooming
facial expression
gesture
space/proximity
listening
volume, prosody, tone, pitch
touch

Interaction Skills
initiation
complimenting
co-operating
turn-taking

Affective Skills
identification of feelings
recognizing own feelings
recognizing feelings of others
trust
disclosures

Cognitive Skills
social perception
self-instruction
self-monitoring evaluation and
  reinforcement
assertion

73. LET'S GO ON A PICNIC

The group members are instructed that they should choose a fellow member with whom they would like to go on a picnic. They should approach that person, saying for example, 'I would like to go on a picnic with you because you are amusing'. The above exercise is then repeated with the following instructions:
'Choose a member who you would like . . .

* to be your mother
* to be your boss
* to be your sister or brother'.

The group reconvenes to discuss their feelings about giving and receiving compliments.

VOICE	LARYNGECTOMY	PHYSICAL DISABILITY	PHONOLOGICAL IMPAIRMENT	MENTAL ILLNESS	HEARING IMPAIRMENT
STUTTER	DYSPHASIA	LEARNING DISABILITY	DYSPRAXIA DYSARTHRIA	ELDERLY	LANGUAGE IMPAIRMENT

Foundation Skills
observation
eye-contact
posture
facial expression
listening
volume, prosody, tone, pitch
memory

Interaction Skills
initiating
listening, responding
termination
co-operating
turn-taking

Affective Skills

Cognitive Skills
social perception
problem solving

---

74. CONSEQUENCES

The group is divided into sub-groups of three and instructed that one member should describe an incident, the second member should give a reason for the incident occurring and the third member should give a possible effect of that incident, e.g. (1)'I got soaked in the rain' (2) 'Because you forgot your umbrella'; (3)'You'll catch a chill'.

VOICE	LARYNGECTOMY	PHYSICAL DISABILITY	PHONOLOGICAL IMPAIRMENT	MENTAL ILLNESS	HEARING IMPAIRMENT
STUTTER	DYSPHASIA	LEARNING DISABILITY	DYSPRAXIA DYSARTHRIA	ELDERLY	LANGUAGE IMPAIRMENT

Foundation Skills
gelling
observation
eye-contact
posture
presentation/grooming
facial expression
gesture
space/proximity
listening
volume, prosody, tone, pitch
touch

Interaction Skills
greetings
initiation
co-operating
turn-taking

Affective Skills
identification of feelings
recognizing own feelings
recognizing feelings of others
trust
disclosures

Cognitive Skills
social perception
self-instruction
self-monitoring evaluation and
 reinforcement
assertion

75. I AM AN OBJECT

The group members are instructed to imagine that they are an object in the room. They should walk around the room and introduce themselves to other group members as this object and name three qualities the object possesses, e.g. 'I am a jumper, I am warm, attractive and feel soft'. The group reconvenes to discuss feelings evoked from making positive statements about oneself.

VOICE	LARYNGECTOMY	**PHYSICAL DISABILITY**	**PHONOLOGICAL IMPAIRMENT**	MENTAL ILLNESS	**HEARING IMPAIRMENT**
STUTTER	DYSPHASIA	**LEARNING DISABILITY**	**DYSPRAXIA DYSARTHRIA**	ELDERLY	**LANGUAGE IMPAIRMENT**

Foundation Skills   **Interaction Skills**
observation   co-operating
posture
facial expression
space/proximity
listening
relaxation

Affective Skills   **Cognitive Skills**
                               self-instruction

76. SLOW MOTION

Group members are instructed to walk round the room as quickly as possible without touching any fellow members. When the leader calls 'Freeze', they are to remain in a static position for a count of five and then start walking in slow motion.

VOICE	LARYNGECTOMY	**PHYSICAL DISABILITY**	**PHONOLOGICAL IMPAIRMENT**	**MENTAL ILLNESS**	**HEARING IMPAIRMENT**
STUTTER	DYSPHASIA	**LEARNING DISABILITY**	**DYSPRAXIA** DYSARTHRIA	ELDERLY	**LANGUAGE IMPAIRMENT**

Foundation Skills
gelling
observation
eye-contact
facial expression
gesture
space/proximity
listening
volume, prosody, tone, pitch
touch
memory

Interaction Skills
greetings
initiation
co-operating
turn-taking

Affective Skills
identification of feelings
recognizing own feelings
recognizing feelings of others
disclosures

Cognitive Skills
assertion

77. LET ME INTRODUCE YOU

The group divides into pairs. Each member should introduce himself by name and make one positive self-statement, e.g. 'I am George and I like playing the piano'. Each pair should seek out another couple and introduce their partner saying his name plus the statement.

VOICE	LARYNGECTOMY	PHYSICAL DISABILITY	PHONOLOGICAL IMPAIRMENT	MENTAL ILLNESS	HEARING IMPAIRMENT
STUTTER	DYSPHASIA	LEARNING DISABILITY	DYSPRAXIA DYSARTHRIA	ELDERLY	LANGUAGE IMPAIRMENT

Foundation Skills   **Interaction Skills**
observation   co-operating
listening   turn-taking
volume, prosody, tone, pitch
touch
memory

Affective Skills   **Cognitive Skills**

78. PASS THE OBJECT

The group is seated in a circle. An article is passed around the group and as each member receives it; he should add to its description, e.g., pencil:

- 'It is blunt'.
- 'It is yellow'.
- 'It is long'.
- 'It doesn't have a rubber'.
- 'It is quite thin'.
- 'It feels smooth'.

VOICE	LARYNGECTOMY	PHYSICAL DISABILITY	PHONOLOGICAL IMPAIRMENT	MENTAL ILLNESS	HEARING IMPAIRMENT
STUTTER	DYSPHASIA	LEARNING DISABILITY	DYSPRAXIA DYSARTHRIA	ELDERLY	LANGUAGE IMPAIRMENT

Foundation Skills   **Interaction Skills**
gelling   co-operation
observation
eye-contact
space/proximity
touch

Affective Skills   **Cognitive Skills**

79. EYE-SWAP CHAIRS

The group members are seated in a circle except one person who stands in the centre of the circle. The seated members are instructed to seek eye-contact with another member and when direct eye-contact is established, they are to change places with each other. Meanwhile, the person standing in the centre is to try to reach an empty chair before the other person.

VOICE	LARYNGECTOMY	PHYSICAL DISABILITY	PHONOLOGICAL IMPAIRMENT	MENTAL ILLNESS	HEARING IMPAIRMENT
STUTTER	DYSPHASIA	LEARNING DISABILITY	DYSPRAXIA DYSARTHRIA	ELDERLY	LANGUAGE IMPAIRMENT

Foundation Skills   **Interaction Skills**
gelling   co-operating
observation   turn-taking
eye-contact
posture
space/proximity
listening (basic)

Affective Skills   **Cognitive Skills**
                                         self-instruction

80. THE BEAR AND THE HONEYPOT

The group is seated on the floor in a circle with one member (the bear)
who is blindfolded being seated in the centre. A 'honeypot', e.g. a box, is
placed next to the bear. The leader points to a member in the circle who
should try to take the honeypot from the bear. The bear should listen
carefully and point to the person who is creeping up on him. If the bear
points correctly, then another person is chosen to steal the honeypot. In
the event that a member is successful in stealing the pot, he changes
places to become the bear and the exercise is repeated.

VOICE	LARYNGECTOMY	**PHYSICAL DISABILITY**	**PHONOLOGICAL IMPAIRMENT**	MENTAL ILLNESS	**HEARING IMPAIRMENT**
STUTTER	DYSPHASIA	**LEARNING DISABILITY**	**DYSPRAXIA** DYSARTHRIA	ELDERLY	**LANGUAGE IMPAIRMENT**

Foundation Skills
gelling
observation
eye-contact
posture
presentation/grooming
facial expression
gesture
space/proximity
listening
memory

Interaction Skills
co-operating
turn-taking

Affective Skills

Cognitive Skills
social perception
problem solving
self-instruction
self-monitoring evaluation
    reinforcement
assertion

81. WHO IS THIS?

The group is seated in a circle. The leader gives a simple physical description of one of the group members, e.g. 'This person has brown hair', 'This person is wearing a red jumper'; 'This person has black shoes'. After each sentence the group is given the opportunity to guess which person is being described. When they have guessed correctly, a new leader is chosen to describe another member. The exercise is repeated until all members have had a turn.

VOICE	LARYNGECTOMY	PHYSICAL DISABILITY	PHONOLOGICAL IMPAIRMENT	MENTAL ILLNESS	HEARING IMPAIRMENT
STUTTER	DYSPHASIA	LEARNING DISABILITY	DYSPRAXIA DYSARTHRIA	ELDERLY	LANGUAGE IMPAIRMENT

Foundation Skills   **Interaction Skills**
gelling   turn-taking

Affective Skills   **Cognitive Skills**
identification of feelings   social perception
recognizing own feelings   self-monitoring evaluation
trust   assertion
disclosures

82. I AM . . .

The group is seated in a circle and is instructed that each member should introduce themselves by stating their name and a fact about themselves which could be either a physical or emotional description, e.g. 'I am Claire; I have brown eyes', or 'I am Joan and I feel very nervous'.

VOICE	LARYNGECTOMY	PHYSICAL DISABILITY	PHONOLOGICAL IMPAIRMENT	MENTAL ILLNESS	HEARING IMPAIRMENT
STUTTER	DYSPHASIA	LEARNING DISABILITY	DYSPRAXIA DYSARTHRIA	ELDERLY	LANGUAGE IMPAIRMENT

Foundation Skills
gelling
observation
eye-contact
facial expression
gesture
space/proximity
listening (basic)
volume, prosody, tone, pitch
memory

Interaction Skills
initiation
topic maintenance
termination
co-operating
turn-taking

Affective Skills

Cognitive Skills
social perception
problem solving
self-instruction
self-monitoring evaluation and
    reinforcement
assertion

83. THE PINK ELEPHANT . . .

The group is divided into pairs. Participants take it in turns to introduce
a topic, e.g. 'Tell me about the pink elephant', or 'Tell me about the
flying saucer'. Their partner should then talk on this topic for up to 30
seconds without stopping. When all group members have had a turn,
the group reconvenes to discuss the skills required to talk about an unfamiliar topic at short notice.

VOICE	LARYNGECTOMY	PHYSICAL DISABILITY	PHONOLOGICAL IMPAIRMENT	MENTAL ILLNESS	HEARING IMPAIRMENT
STUTTER	DYSPHASIA	LEARNING DISABILITY	DYSPRAXIA DYSARTHRIA	ELDERLY	LANGUAGE IMPAIRMENT

Foundation Skills
gelling
observation
eye-contact
posture
facial expression
gesture
space/proximity
listening
volume, prosody, tone, pitch
touch
memory

Interaction Skills
initiation
listening/reflecting back, responding
topic maintenance/repair of
    conversations
termination
co-operating
turn-taking, breaking in, interrupting

Affective Skills

Cognitive Skills
social perception
problem solving
self-instruction
self-monitoring evaluation and
    reinforcement
negotiating
assertion

84. LOOK AT THE PICTURE

The group is divided into pairs and given a picture of an activity, e.g. a shopping scene. One member is to talk about the picture whilst their partner is to interrupt, e.g.:

* *Partner A:* 'There is a supermarket in the picture and the man has brought a loaf of bread. The shopping trolley is empty and the lady is putting her shopping in her bag'.
* *Partner B:*   will interrupt during the talk, e.g.: 'What about that baby in the pram?'

Partner A will need to respond and then continue. Roles should then be reversed. The group reconvenes to discuss interruptions and strategies for repair of conversation.

VOICE	LARYNGECTOMY	**PHYSICAL DISABILITY**	**PHONOLOGICAL IMPAIRMENT**	**MENTAL ILLNESS**	**HEARING IMPAIRMENT**
STUTTER	**DYSPHASIA**	**LEARNING DISABILITY**	**DYSPRAXIA DYSARTHRIA**	**ELDERLY**	**LANGUAGE IMPAIRMENT**

Foundation Skills   **Interaction Skills**
listening   co-operating
memory   turn-taking

Affective Skills   **Cognitive Skills**
                               social perception
                               problem solving
                               self-instruction
                               self-monitoring

85. I AM GOING TO THE MOON

The group sits in a circle and the leader explains that they will say the
following sentence: 'My name is Sally, I am going to the moon and I am
taking a sun hat with me'. The group members each have a turn saying
the same sentence using their own name and an object. They are to
discover the 'rule' of the exercise which is that they can only take something with them that begins with the same letter as their name. The exercise is completed when everyone has discovered the rule and is
'allowed' to take their object to the moon.

Modification
To simplify:
* Reduce the length and complexity of the sentence, e.g. 'I am *M*ary, I
  like *m*armalade'.

VOICE	LARYNGECTOMY	**PHYSICAL DISABILITY**	**PHONOLOGICAL IMPAIRMENT**	**MENTAL ILLNESS**	**HEARING IMPAIRMENT**
STUTTER	**DYSPHASIA**	**LEARNING DISABILITY**	**DYSPRAXIA DYSARTHRIA**	**ELDERLY**	**LANGUAGE IMPAIRMENT**

Foundation Skills
observation
eye-contact
posture
facial expression
gesture
space/proximity
listening (basic)
volume, prosody, tone, pitch
touch
memory

Interaction Skills
initiating/asking questions
listening/reflecting back, responding
answering questions/responding
topic maintenance/repair of
    conversations
termination
complimenting
co-operating
turn-taking

Affective Skills
identification of feelings
recognizing own feelings
recognizing feelings of others
trust
disclosures

Cognitive Skills
social perception
problem solving
self-instruction
self-monitoring evaluation and
    reinforcement
negotiating
assertion

86. SHIPWRECKED

The group is divided into sub-groups of four members. They are instructed that they are to imagine that they are stranded on a raft in the ocean following a shipwreck. In order for the raft to remain afloat, only three people may remain aboard. The sub-group is to negotiate for 5 – 7 minutes which member will have to leave the raft. At the end of the allotted time, the group re-forms to discuss their feelings and how the negotiation took place.

VOICE	LARYNGECTOMY	PHYSICAL DISABILITY	PHONOLOGICAL IMPAIRMENT	MENTAL ILLNESS	HEARING IMPAIRMENT
STUTTER	DYSPHASIA	LEARNING DISABILITY	DYSPRAXIA DYSARTHRIA	ELDERLY	LANGUAGE IMPAIRMENT

Foundation Skills
observation
eye-contact
posture
presentation/grooming
facial expression
gesture
space/proximity
listening
volume, prosody, tone, pitch

Interaction Skills
complimenting
co-operating
turn-taking

Affective Skills
identification of feelings
recognizing own feelings
trust
disclosures

Cognitive Skills
social perception
self-monitoring evaluation and
    reinforcement
assertion

87. DO I LOOK GOOD?

The group is divided into pairs and they are given one minute to say one positive and one negative statement about their partner's appearance. The group re-forms to discuss presentation and grooming of self as well as their feelings regarding positive and negative statements.

VOICE	LARYNGECTOMY	PHYSICAL DISABILITY	PHONOLOGICAL IMPAIRMENT	MENTAL ILLNESS	HEARING IMPAIRMENT
STUTTER	DYSPHASIA	LEARNING DISABILITY	DYSPRAXIA DYSARTHRIA	ELDERLY	LANGUAGE IMPAIRMENT

Foundation Skills
observation
eye-contact
posture
facial expression
gesture
space/proximity
listening
volume, prosody, tone, pitch
memory

Interaction Skills
listening, responding
co-operating
turn-taking

Affective Skills
identification of feelings
recognizing own feelings
recognizing feelings of others

Cognitive Skills
social perception
self-instruction
self-monitoring evaluation

88. EMOTIONAL NURSERY RHYMES

A selection of cards is prepared, each with a different emotion written on it, e.g. bored, disappointed, happy. One card is given to each group member and the group is instructed to divide into pairs. The pairs are seated opposite one another and each person must recite a nursery rhyme in a manner which depicts the emotion written on their card, using appropriate facial expression, gesture and intonation. Their partner is then required to guess what the emotion is. When each member has taken a turn at the exercise, the group re-forms to discuss how emotions are shown, both verbally and non-verbally.

Modifications
To simplify:
• Sentences or phrases may be used instead of nursery rhymes.
• Pictures may be used to demonstrate the different emotions.

VOICE	LARYNGECTOMY	PHYSICAL DISABILITY	PHONOLOGICAL IMPAIRMENT	MENTAL ILLNESS	HEARING IMPAIRMENT
STUTTER	DYSPHASIA	LEARNING DISABILITY	DYSPRAXIA DYSARTHRIA	ELDERLY	LANGUAGE IMPAIRMENT

Foundation Skills
observation
eye-contact
posture
facial expression
gesture
space/proximity

Interaction Skills
co-operating

Affective Skills
trust

Cognitive Skills

89. SHADOWS

The group is divided into pairs who stand opposite each other. One person should be the leader whilst his partner will be the shadow. The leader performs an action, e.g. combing his hair. He should move slowly to allow his shadow to maintain eye-contact and mirror the movements of the leader exactly. Roles should then be reversed.

Modifications

To simplify:
- The leader may suggest body movements and actions.
- One static posture to be shadowed rather than a moving action.

VOICE	LARYNGECTOMY	PHYSICAL DISABILITY	**PHONOLOGICAL IMPAIRMENT**	**MENTAL ILLNESS**	**HEARING IMPAIRMENT**
STUTTER	DYSPHASIA	**LEARNING DISABILITY**	**DYSPRAXIA DYSARTHRIA**	ELDERLY	**LANGUAGE IMPAIRMENT**

Foundation Skills   **Interaction Skills**
gelling   co-operating
observation
eye-contact
posture
facial expression
listening
memory

Affective Skills   **Cognitive Skills**
                              problem solving
                              self-monitoring, evaluation and
                                  reinforcement

90. YOU'RE GETTING THERE

The leader explains that one person will leave the room while the rest of the group decide on a posture that they would like that person to adopt. They will guide the person towards the desired posture by clapping. A volunteer then leaves the room and the group select the posture, e.g. stand on one leg, sit on the floor. The member is invited back into the room and the group guides him by frequency and loudness of clapping until he achieves the desired posture.

Modifications
To simplify:
• Pictures of postures are used. The member leaves the room whilst the rest of the group chooses a picture from a selection of four. The member then returns to the room, is shown all four pictures and then chooses to take up one of the postures. If correct, the group applauds, if incorrect he is instructed to try an alternative.

Limited mobility:
• Instead of a posture, choose a location in the room as the desired goal; a helper assists the member around the room, guided by clapping until they reach the desired place.

VOICE	LARYNGECTOMY	**PHYSICAL DISABILITY**	**PHONOLOGICAL IMPAIRMENT**	MENTAL ILLNESS	**HEARING IMPAIRMENT**
STUTTER	DYSPHASIA	**LEARNING DISABILITY**	**DYSPRAXIA** DYSARTHRIA	ELDERLY	**LANGUAGE IMPAIRMENT**

Foundation Skills   **Interaction Skills**
gelling   co-operating
space/proximity
touch

Affective Skills   **Cognitive Skills**
                               assertion

91. THE NEWSPAPER GAME

The group is divided into sub-groups of three and each sub-group is given a large sheet of newspaper, e.g. *The Times*. They are instructed to place the newspaper on the floor and all the members of the sub-group should stand on it, with nobody standing over the edge. When this has been achieved, they are instructed to step off the newspaper, fold the sheet in half and then all stand on it. The exercise continues until it is no longer possible for all members to be standing on the paper. The large group re-forms to discuss their feelings regarding proximity and touch.

VOICE	LARYNGECTOMY	PHYSICAL DISABILITY	PHONOLOGICAL IMPAIRMENT	MENTAL ILLNESS	HEARING IMPAIRMENT
STUTTER	DYSPHASIA	LEARNING DISABILITY	DYSPRAXIA DYSARTHRIA	ELDERLY	LANGUAGE IMPAIRMENT

Foundation Skills	Interaction Skills
observation	responding
eye-contact	co-operating
listening	turn-taking
memory	

Affective Skills	Cognitive Skills
	self-instruction

92. SAY THREE WORDS

The group is seated in a circle with a leader in the centre. The leader's eyes should be closed whilst a ball is passed around the circle. The leader then claps, opens her eyes and calls out a letter of the alphabet. The group member who is holding the ball should then say three words beginning with that letter. The exercise should be repeated with a different letter.

Modification
To simplify:
• Reduce the number of words to be said by the person holding the ball.

VOICE	LARYNGECTOMY	**PHYSICAL DISABILITY**	**PHONOLOGICAL IMPAIRMENT**	**MENTAL ILLNESS**	**HEARING IMPAIRMENT**
STUTTER	DYSPHASIA	**LEARNING DISABILITY**	**DYSPRAXIA** DYSARTHRIA	**ELDERLY**	**LANGUAGE IMPAIRMENT**

Foundation Skills
eye-contact
posture
facial expression
gelling
listening (basic)

Interaction Skills
listening
turn-taking
complimenting
co-operating
responding

Affective Skills
identification of feelings
recognizing own feelings
recognizing feelings of others
trust

Cognitive Skills
social perception
assertion
self-monitoring

---

93. PRAISE PARCELS

The group is divided into pairs. Each member is instructed to write down a compliment for their partner. They are then asked to fold their piece of paper into a parcel and give it to their partner who is to read the compliment aloud and respond appropriately. When each member has had a turn, the group discusses feelings related to giving and receiving compliments.

VOICE	LARYNGECTOMY	PHYSICAL DISABILITY	PHONOLOGICAL IMPAIRMENT	MENTAL ILLNESS	HEARING IMPAIRMENT
STUTTER	DYSPHASIA	LEARNING DISABILITY	DYSPRAXIA DYSARTHRIA	ELDERLY	LANGUAGE IMPAIRMENT

Foundation Skills
gelling
observation
eye-contact
posture
presentation/grooming/facial expression
gesture
space proximity
listening
volume, prosody, tone, pitch
touch
memory

Interaction Skills
co-operating
listening
turn-taking
responding

Affective Skills
identification of feelings
recognizing own feelings
recognizing feelings of others
trust
disclosures

Cognitive Skills
social perception
self-instruction
self-monitoring
assertion

94. ARRANGE YOURSELVES

The group is instructed to choose a social situation, for example, a party or a meeting at work, and are asked to illustrate the social situation by arranging themselves in the room as they would like to be in that social setting. The exercise is to be carried out without talking. When all group members are in place they are to remain in that position for 30 seconds. The group then re-forms to discuss feelings evoked from carrying out the exercise.

VOICE	LARYNGECTOMY	PHYSICAL DISABILITY	PHONOLOGICAL IMPAIRMENT	MENTAL ILLNESS	HEARING IMPAIRMENT
STUTTER	DYSPHASIA	LEARNING DISABILITY	DYSPRAXIA DYSARTHRIA	ELDERLY	LANGUAGE IMPAIRMENT

Foundation Skills	Interaction Skills
gelling	greeting
listening	initiation
eye-contact	termination
facial expression	turn-taking

Affective Skills	Cognitive Skills

95. MEET MY NEIGHBOUR

The group is seated in a circle, each member wearing a label with their name clearly printed on it. Each group member is asked to introduce the person on their left by saying their name and making up a short story about them, e.g. 'This is John and John is a bit tired today because he's just come back from walking to the North Pole'. This continues until all members have been introduced.

VOICE	LARYNGECTOMY	PHYSICAL DISABILITY	PHONOLOGICAL IMPAIRMENT	MENTAL ILLNESS	HEARING IMPAIRMENT
STUTTER	DYSPHASIA	LEARNING DISABILITY	DYSPRAXIA DYSARTHRIA	ELDERLY	LANGUAGE IMPAIRMENT

Foundation Skills   **Interaction Skills**
gelling   listening
listening   initiation
eye-contact   termination
facial expression   topic maintenance
posture
gesture
memory

Affective Skills   **Cognitive Skills**
                               problem solving
                               self-monitoring

96. TELL ME A STORY

A selection of cards is prepared, each with a different story title written on it, e.g. *The Party*, or *The Tale of the Three Farmers*. The group is divided into pairs, each member being seated opposite their partner. One card is given to each group member and each person is given 30 seconds to make up a story based on the title on their card. When all group members have had a turn, the group reconvenes to discuss the skills required to generate a story at short notice.

VOICE	LARYNGECTOMY	PHYSICAL DISABILITY	PHONOLOGICAL IMPAIRMENT	MENTAL ILLNESS	HEARING IMPAIRMENT
STUTTER	DYSPHASIA	LEARNING DISABILITY	DYSPRAXIA DYSARTHRIA	**ELDERLY**	LANGUAGE IMPAIRMENT

Foundation Skills   **Interaction Skills**
gelling   topic maintenance
listening   initiation
eye-contact   termination
facial expression   turn-taking
volume, prosody, tone, pitch

Affective Skills   **Cognitive Skills**
                                         problem solving
                                         self-instruction
                                         self-monitoring

97. LUCKY DIP STORY TELLING

The group is divided into pairs and each pair is given a bag containing an assortment of objects. The pairs are instructed to take it in turns to pull out three items from the bag and to make up a story which includes each of the items picked out. The exercise continues until each group member has generated a story. The group re-forms to discuss the skills required to generate a story from three items.

VOICE	LARYNGECTOMY	PHYSICAL DISABILITY	PHONOLOGICAL IMPAIRMENT	MENTAL ILLNESS	HEARING IMPAIRMENT
STUTTER	DYSPHASIA	LEARNING DISABILITY	DYSPRAXIA DYSARTHRIA	ELDERLY	LANGUAGE IMPAIRMENT

Foundation Skills
gelling
listening
eye-contact
observation
memory
gesture
space

Interaction Skills
responding
initiation
co-operating

Affective Skills
disclosure

Cognitive Skills
problem solving
negotiating
assertion

98. IN A LINE

The group members are instructed to organize themselves into a line according to criteria given by the leader. For example, the person with the longest hair to be at the front of the line and the person with the shortest hair at the back, or the person living the closest to the group's venue to be at the front and the person living furthest away from the venue at the back. When a line has been formed the group members reassemble to discuss what skills were involved in arranging themselves into a line.

VOICE	LARYNGECTOMY	PHYSICAL DISABILITY	PHONOLOGICAL IMPAIRMENT	MENTAL ILLNESS	HEARING IMPAIRMENT
STUTTER	DYSPHASIA	LEARNING DISABILITY	DYSPRAXIA DYSARTHRIA	ELDERLY	LANGUAGE IMPAIRMENT

Foundation Skills   **Interaction Skills**
gelling
listening
memory
volume, prosody, tone, pitch

Affective Skills   **Cognitive Skills**

99. THE BLINDFOLD GAME

The group is seated in a circle. The leader blindfolds a group member
and then points to another member in the circle who is to say 'Hello . . .'
to the blindfolded person. The remainder of the group are to remain
quiet whilst the blindfolded member listens carefully and names the
person who has spoken. The exercise is repeated until all members have
had a turn at being blindfolded.

VOICE	LARYNGECTOMY	**PHYSICAL DISABILITY**	**PHONOLOGICAL IMPAIRMENT**	**MENTAL ILLNESS**	HEARING IMPAIRMENT
STUTTER	**DYSPHASIA**	**LEARNING DISABILITY**	**DYSPRAXIA DYSARTHRIA**	**ELDERLY**	**LANGUAGE IMPAIRMENT**

Foundation Skills   **Interaction Skills**
gelling
observation
eye-contact
facial expression
gesture
listening

Affective Skills   **Cognitive Skills**
identification of feelings
recognizing own feelings
recognizing feelings of others
trust
disclosures

---

100. POSTCARDS

The group is seated in a circle. The group members are asked to arrange a large range of cards/postcards in the centre of the circle and instructed to find three cards which depict how they are feeling. When each group member has chosen three pictures they are given the opportunity to discuss their choice.

VOICE	LARYNGECTOMY	PHYSICAL DISABILITY	PHONOLOGICAL IMPAIRMENT	MENTAL ILLNESS	HEARING IMPAIRMENT
STUTTER	DYSPHASIA	LEARNING DISABILITY	DYSPRAXIA DYSARTHRIA	ELDERLY	LANGUAGE IMPAIRMENT

Foundation Skills   **Interaction Skills**
gelling
gesture
posture
facial expression
listening
observation
eye-contact

Affective Skills   **Cognitive Skills**
                                         problem solving

---

101. SPOT THE RULE

The group is seated in a circle. The leader informs the group that the activity will begin with the leader modelling a sentence, e.g. 'I am going to take a train from ... to ...'. The person seated to the leader's left is then to repeat the sentence but choose two different destinations. The group leader will have generated a rule which determines whether the two destinations chosen are acceptable or not. The aim of the activity is for the group members to identify this rule. The rule can be changed according to which social skill is being worked on. For example, a response is only acceptable if the two destinations chosen begin with adjacent letters of the alphabet or if an 'um' is inserted before naming the second destination or if arms are crossed prior to repeating the phrase.

VOICE	LARYNGECTOMY	PHYSICAL DISABILITY	PHONOLOGICAL IMPAIRMENT	MENTAL ILLNESS	HEARING IMPAIRMENT
STUTTER	DYSPHASIA	LEARNING DISABILITY	DYSPRAXIA DYSARTHRIA	ELDERLY	LANGUAGE IMPAIRMENT

Foundation Skills   **Interaction Skills**
gelling
observation
eye-contact
facial expression
gesture
space proximity
touch

Affective Skills   **Cognitive Skills**

102. DRAW IT

The group is divided into pairs. One member of each pair is given a simple line drawing of a scene, for example, a house next to a tree with a sun in the sky. Using gesture and without talking, the client shows their partner how to draw the scene. The person who is drawing should only carry out the instructions given by their partner. When the task is completed roles should be reversed. The group then re-forms to discuss strategies used to give instructions non-verbally.

VOICE	LARYNGECTOMY	PHYSICAL DISABILITY	**PHONOLOGICAL IMPAIRMENT**	**MENTAL ILLNESS**	**HEARING IMPAIRMENT**
STUTTER	DYSPHASIA	**LEARNING DISABILITY**	**DYSPRAXIA** DYSARTHRIA	ELDERLY	**LANGUAGE IMPAIRMENT**

Foundation Skills   **Interaction Skills**
gelling   listening
observation   turn-taking
posture
facial expression
gesture
listening
memory

Affective Skills   **Cognitive Skills**
identification of feelings
recognizing own feelings
recognizing feelings of others
trust
disclosures

103. SOUND AND MOVEMENT

The group stands in a circle. The leader begins the activity by producing
a movement, accompanied by a sound which illustrates how they are
feeling. For example, jumping in the air with a 'whoosh' sound, or
tapping your feet slowly with a 'bleep bleep' sound. Members are then
instructed as a group to repeat the sound and movement. The activity
continues until each group member has had a turn at producing their
own sound and movement. Group members should then be given the
opportunity to comment on their choices of sound and movement and
the feelings evoked from carrying out the activity.

VOICE	LARYNGECTOMY	**PHYSICAL DISABILITY**	**PHONOLOGICAL IMPAIRMENT**	**MENTAL ILLNESS**	**HEARING IMPAIRMENT**
STUTTER	DYSPHASIA	**LEARNING DISABILITY**	**DYSPRAXIA** DYSARTHRIA	**ELDERLY**	**LANGUAGE IMPAIRMENT**

Foundation Skills   **Interaction Skills**
eye-contact
space/proximity
listening
volume, tone, prosody, pitch
memory
gelling

Affective Skills   **Cognitive Skills**

104. SPIN THE PLATE

The group is seated in a circle. One member is selected to stand in the centre of the circle and their chair is removed. The person standing in the centre is instructed to spin a plate and call out the name of another group member. The named group member attempts to catch the spinning plate before it stops spinning and the person standing in the centre sits on the empty chair. The activity continues until all members have been given at least one turn at spinning the plate.

VOICE	LARYNGECTOMY	PHYSICAL DISABILITY	**PHONOLOGICAL IMPAIRMENT**	**MENTAL ILLNESS**	**HEARING IMPAIRMENT**
STUTTER	DYSPHASIA	**LEARNING DISABILITY**	DYSPRAXIA DYSARTHRIA	ELDERLY	**LANGUAGE IMPAIRMENT**

Foundation Skills
volume, prosody, tone, pitch
eye-contact
listening
facial expression
gesture
posture
space/proximity

Interaction Skills
co-operating

Affective Skills
identification of feelings

Cognitive Skills
self-instruction
assertion

105. THE 'DON'T LISTEN' EXERCISE

The group is divided into pairs and seated opposite each other. One member of the pair is selected to be a speaker and the other member a listener. The speaker is instructed to give a short, simple account of an event which actually happened to him. The listener is instructed actively *not* to listen to what is said. The exercise is repeated until each person has adopted both a speaker and listener role. The group reassembles to discuss listening and the effects of not being listened to.

VOICE	LARYNGECTOMY	PHYSICAL DISABILITY	PHONOLOGICAL IMPAIRMENT	MENTAL ILLNESS	HEARING IMPAIRMENT
STUTTER	DYSPHASIA	LEARNING DISABILITY	DYSPRAXIA DYSARTHRIA	ELDERLY	LANGUAGE IMPAIRMENT

Foundation Skills
posture
listening
eye-contact
facial expression
space/proximity
gesture
volume, prosody, tone, pitch
memory

Interaction Skills
listening
initiation
responding
co-operating
complimenting

Affective Skills
recognizing own feelings
recognizing feelings of others

Cognitive Skills
problem solving
self-instruction
self-monitoring
negotiating
assertion

106. PERSUASION

The group is divided into pairs. One member is chosen to sit down on a chair and their partner to stand up. The person standing up is given two minutes to persuade the person sitting down to give up his chair. The person doing the persuading is instructed to use a range of strategies apart from physical violence. After two minutes, roles are reversed. The group re-forms to discuss feelings evoked in the different roles.

VOICE	LARYNGECTOMY	PHYSICAL DISABILITY	PHONOLOGICAL IMPAIRMENT	MENTAL ILLNESS	HEARING IMPAIRMENT
STUTTER	DYSPHASIA	LEARNING DISABILITY	DYSPRAXIA DYSARTHRIA	ELDERLY	LANGUAGE IMPAIRMENT

Foundation Skills	Interaction Skills
posture	answering/responding
listening	initiation
eye-contact	co-operating
facial expression	complimenting
gelling	
observation	
volume, prosody, tone, pitch	
memory	

Affective Skills	Cognitive Skills
recognizing own feelings	
recognizing feelings of others	
disclosure	

107. IMAGINARY GIFTS

The group is seated in a circle. The leader instructs the group that each member in turn is to think of an imaginary gift to give to the person sitting on their left. Group members are encouraged to choose a gift that is particularly relevant to the person. For example, one person may choose a camera because the person sitting to their left is about to go on a safari holiday. The leader should start the exercise and when each member has had a turn the group should be given the opportunity to discuss their choice and the feelings evoked from receiving an imaginary gift.

VOICE	LARYNGECTOMY	PHYSICAL DISABILITY	PHONOLOGICAL IMPAIRMENT	MENTAL ILLNESS	HEARING IMPAIRMENT
STUTTER	DYSPHASIA	LEARNING DISABILITY	DYSPRAXIA DYSARTHRIA	ELDERLY	LANGUAGE IMPAIRMENT

Foundation Skills
posture
listening
eye-contact
facial expression
gelling
gesture
space (proximity)
touch

Interaction Skills
co-operating

Affective Skills

Cognitive Skills
self-instruction

108. STROKE THE CAT

The group is divided into pairs. One member is chosen to crouch on the floor and pretend to be a cat and their partner is the cat owner. The cat owner is instructed to stroke the cat and is timed to see how long they are able to keep stroking the cat without showing any signs of laughing. If the cat owner laughs, then roles are reversed. The activity continues until all group members have had a turn at being a cat and a cat owner. The group reassembles to discuss the difficulties with not laughing.

VOICE	LARYNGECTOMY	PHYSICAL DISABILITY	**PHONOLOGICAL IMPAIRMENT**	MENTAL ILLNESS	**HEARING IMPAIRMENT**
STUTTER	DYSPHASIA	**LEARNING DISABILITY**	**DYSPRAXIA** DYSARTHRIA	ELDERLY	**LANGUAGE IMPAIRMENT**

Foundation Skills   **Interaction Skills**
gelling
listening
gesture
facial expression

Affective Skills   **Cognitive Skills**

109. BLIND MAN'S BUFF

The group stands in a circle with one group member who is blindfolded standing in the middle. The leader points to two group members standing on opposite sides of the circle, who are to attempt to change places with each other. The person standing in the middle should listen carefully and try to catch a group member before they manage to change places. If a group member is caught, the exercise begins again with the leader choosing two different group members to change places with each other. In the event that the two group members are successful at changing placcs, then another person is chosen to be blindfolded.

VOICE	LARYNGECTOMY	PHYSICAL DISABILITY	**PHONOLOGICAL IMPAIRMENT**	MENTAL ILLNESS	**HEARING IMPAIRMENT**
STUTTER	DYSPHASIA	**LEARNING DISABILITY**	**DYSPRAXIA DYSARTHRIA**	ELDERLY	**LANGUAGE IMPAIRMENT**

Foundation Skills	**Interaction Skills**
gelling	turn-taking
listening	
eye-contact	
volume	

Affective Skills	**Cognitive Skills**

110. ANIMAL, VEGETABLE AND MINERAL

The group stands in a circle. The leader begins the exercise by passing or throwing a ball to another group member and calling out either 'animal', 'vegetable', or 'mineral'. If the word 'animal', is called out, the group member catching the ball must call out the name of an animal, before passing the ball on to another group member. Similarly, if the word 'vegetable' is called out, the name of a vegetable needs to be given and a mineral if the word 'mineral' is called out. The exercise continues until all group members have had at least one turn at throwing the ball.

VOICE	LARYNGECTOMY	PHYSICAL DISABILITY	PHONOLOGICAL IMPAIRMENT	MENTAL ILLNESS	HEARING IMPAIRMENT
STUTTER	DYSPHASIA	LEARNING DISABILITY	DYSPRAXIA DYSARTHRIA	ELDERLY	LANGUAGE IMPAIRMENT

Foundation Skills   **Interaction Skills**
gelling
observation
memory

Affective Skills   **Cognitive Skills**
                              self-monitoring

111. REMEMBER THE PICTURE

The group is divided into sub-groups of three. Each sub-group is shown
a photograph of an advertisement from a magazine and is instructed that
they have one minute to study the picture carefully. The photograph or
advertisement is then taken away and group members are asked to recall
as many items as they can remember from the picture.

VOICE	LARYNGECTOMY	PHYSICAL DISABILITY	PHONOLOGICAL IMPAIRMENT	MENTAL ILLNESS	HEARING IMPAIRMENT
STUTTER	DYSPHASIA	LEARNING DISABILITY	DYSPRAXIA DYSARTHRIA	ELDERLY	LANGUAGE IMPAIRMENT

Foundation Skills	Interaction Skills
gelling	turn-taking
observation	
eye-contact	
volume	
facial expression	
memory	
listening	

Affective Skills	Cognitive Skills
	self-instruction
	self-monitoring

112. HELLO HARRY

The group is seated in a circle on the floor. The leader begins the exercises by turning to the person sitting on their left and saying, 'Hello Harry, call Harry'. The person sitting to the left of the leader is then to turn to the person on their left and repeat the phrase, 'Hello Harry, call Harry' and so on around the circle. The aim of the activity is for group members to maintain a blank facial expression and not laugh whilst saying the phrase. If a group member laughs they are given a sticker which is stuck on their face. They will now be addressed as 'One spot' rather than 'Harry', and not laugh.

VOICE	LARYNGECTOMY	PHYSICAL DISABILITY	PHONOLOGICAL IMPAIRMENT	MENTAL ILLNESS	HEARING IMPAIRMENT
STUTTER	DYSPHASIA	LEARNING DISABILITY	DYSPRAXIA DYSARTHRIA	ELDERLY	LANGUAGE IMPAIRMENT

Foundation Skills	**Interaction Skills**
gelling	complimenting
volume	co-operating
memory	
facial expression	

Affective Skills	**Cognitive Skills**
	assertion

113. GOOD NEWS SOUND

Each member of the group states his name preceded with a positive adjective starting with the same initial sound as the person's name. The word might be an -ing word that describes something the person does well or it might be a descriptive adjective, e.g. singing Sarah, or generous George.

VOICE	LARYNGECTOMY	PHYSICAL DISABILITY	PHONOLOGICAL IMPAIRMENT	MENTAL ILLNESS	HEARING IMPAIRMENT
STUTTER	DYSPHASIA	LEARNING DISABILITY	DYSPRAXIA DYSARTHRIA	ELDERLY	LANGUAGE IMPAIRMENT

Appendix
Chart for Practical
Achivities

Patient Group: Voice

EXERCISE NUMBER:	1	2	3	4	5	6	7	8	9	10	11	12	13	14	15	16	17	18	19	20	21	22	23	24	25	26	27	28	29	30	31	32	33	34	35	36	37
Foundation skills																																					
Gelling											o									o				o	o	o	o	o	o			o	o		o	o	
Observation	o										o									o				o	o	o	o	o	o			o	o		o	o	o
Eye-contact	o										o									o				o	o	o	o	o	o			o	o		o		o
Posture																								o	o	o											
Presentation/grooming																		o	o																		
Facial expression											o							o		o				o	o	o	o					o	o		o	o	o
Gesture	o				o													o		o				o				o					o	o		o	
Space/proximity	o										o									o				o	o							o	o			o	
Listening (basic)	o										o							o		o				o		o	o					o	o			o	
Volume, prosody, etc	o										o							o		o				o												o	o
Relaxation																									o												
Touch																								o			o	o									
Memory	o										o							o		o				o	o	o		o	o								
Interaction skills																																					
Greetings											o									o				o	o				o				o			o	
Initiation/asking											o									o					o				o								
Listening (advanced)	o										o									o							o		o								
Answering/responding											o									o									o								
Topic maintenance																				o									o								
Termination	o										o																		o								
Complimenting																													o								
Co-operating											o							o		o				o		o	o	o	o			o	o		o	o	
Turn-taking, breaking in	o										o							o		o				o	o	o	o	o	o			o	o		o	o	
Affective skills																																					
Identification of feelings																		o		o						o	o	o	o			o	o		o	o	
Recognizing own feelings																		o		o						o	o	o	o			o	o		o		
other's feelings																				o								o	o			o					
Trust																		o										o	o								
Disclosures	o									o								o								o		o	o								
Cognitive skills																																					
Social perception																		o		o				o	o	o	o	o	o			o	o		o	o	
Problem-solving																									o	o	o	o									
Self-instruction																		o		o																	
Self-monitoring, etc.	o																	o		o									o			o	o			o	
Negotiating																								o					o								
Assertion																													o								

Patient Group: Voice (contd)

EXERCISE NUMBER:	38	39	40	41	42	43	44	45	46	47	48	49	50	51	52	53	54	55	56	57	58	59	60	61	62	63	64	65	66	67	68	69	70	71	72	73	74
Foundation skills																																					
Gelling																				57				○			○				○	○	○	○	○	○	○
Observation	○	○	○					○		○					○		○	○		○				○		○	○			○	○	○	○	○	○	○	○
Eye-contact	○	○	○					○		○					○		○	○		○				○		○				○	○	○	○	○	○	○	○
Posture								○		○							○	○						○							○	○	○	○	○	○	○
Presentation/grooming																																					
Facial expression	○	○	○					○		○					○		○	○		○		○		○		○				○	○	○	○	○	○	○	○
Gesture	○	○	○					○		○							○					○		○		○	○			○	○	○	○	○	○	○	○
Space/proximity	○	○						○		○																					○	○	○	○			
Listening (basic)	○	○	○					○		○			○		○		○	○	○			○		○		○				○	○	○					
Volume, prosody, etc	○	○						○		○			○		○		○	○	○	○		○		○		○				○	○						
Relaxation																											○										
Touch								○		○							○			○		○		○		○				○	○	○	○		○		○
Memory			○					○		○			○				○		○																		
Interaction skills																																					
Greetings																															○	○			○	○	
Initiation/asking																															○	○	○	○	○	○	○
Listening (advanced)																								○							○	○	○		○	○	○
Answering/responding																		○	○												○	○					
Topic maintenance																		○	○												○	○	○				
Termination																																					
Complimenting	○							○		○							○	○	○		○			○		○	○			○	○	○	○		○	○	○
Co-operating								○		○			○				○	○	○		○			○		○	○			○	○	○	○		○	○	○
Turn-taking, breaking in																																					
Affective skills																																					
Identification of feelings	○	○																						○		○				○	○	○	○		○	○	○
Recognizing own feelings																			○					○		○					○	○					
other's feelings	○																		○							○				○	○	○					
Trust																			○							○				○	○	○					
Disclosures																			○							○											
Cognitive skills																																					
Social perception	○														○									○		○				○	○	○	○		○		○
Problem-solving	○											○			○				○					○							○	○	○				
Self-instruction																			○												○	○	○				
Self-monitoring, etc.																										○					○	○					
Negotiating																			○																○	○	
Assertion																										○					○				○		○

Patient Group: Voice (contd)

EXERCISE NUMBER:	75	76	77	78	79	80	81	82	83	84	85	86	87	88	89	90	91	92	93	94	95	96	97	98	99	100	101	102	103	104	105	106	107	108	109	110	111	112	113
Foundation skills																																							
Gelling	o							o	o											o			o	o		o	o					o	o						
Observation	o							o	o					o						o			o	o		o	o					o	o		o	o	o	o	
Eye-contact	o							o	o			o	o	o	o					o			o			o	o					o	o	o					
Posture											o	o	o	o	o				o	o			o			o													
Presentation/grooming													o																										
Facial expression	o							o				o	o	o	o					o			o			o	o			o	o	o	o		o				
Gesture	o							o				o	o	o	o					o						o	o			o	o	o							
Space/proximity	o							o				o	o	o			o			o			o			o				o	o	o							
Listening (basic)	o							o				o	o	o						o			o			o	o			o	o	o	o		o	o	o	o	
Volume, prosody, etc	o							o				o	o	o						o			o	o		o				o	o	o	o		o	o	o	o	
Relaxation																																							
Touch	o											o				o				o																			
Memory	o					o		o				o	o	o						o		o	o	o							o	o					o	o	o
Interaction skills																																							
Greetings	o											o	o								o										o	o							
Initiation/asking	o							o				o	o	o						o	o	o		o						o	o	o							
Listening (advanced)												o		o						o										o	o	o							
Answering/responding									o			o							o			o	o																
Topic maintenance									o			o							o			o	o																
Termination												o																											
Complimenting												o	o	o						o				o						o	o	o	o						
Co-operating	o							o	o			o	o	o				o		o			o							o	o	o	o						
Turn-taking, breaking in	o							o	o			o	o	o						o													o						
Affective skills																																							
Identification of feelings	o							o				o	o	o			o			o						o				o		o							
Recognizing own feelings	o							o				o	o	o						o						o				o	o		o						
other's feelings	o											o	o	o						o						o				o	o								
Trust								o				o	o	o						o						o						o							
Disclosures	o							o				o	o	o	o					o				o								o							
Cognitive skills																																							
Social perception								o				o	o				o			o			o	o								o							
Problem-solving								o				o	o							o			o	o		o						o							
Self-instruction						o		o				o	o	o						o			o	o						o	o	o				o			
Self-monitoring, etc.								o				o	o	o						o			o	o						o	o	o							
Negotiating								o				o								o																			
Assertion	o							o				o	o	o																									o

Patient Group: Laryngectomy

EXERCISE NUMBER:	1	2	3	4	5	6	7	8	9	10	11	12	13	14	15	16	17	18	19	20	21	22	23	24	25	26	27	28	29	30	31	32	33	34	35	36	37
Foundation skills																																					
Gelling		o	o								o									o				o	o	o	o	o	o			o	o	o	o	o	
Observation		o	o																	o	o			o	o	o	o	o	o			o	o	o	o	o	
Eye-contact	o		o							o	o									o	o			o	o	o	o	o	o			o	o	o	o	o	
Posture	o									o	o									o	o			o		o	o	o	o				o	o			
Presentation/grooming	o																																				
Facial expression	o										o							o	o	o	o	o		o	o	o	o		o			o	o	o	o	o	
Gesture	o		o								o							o	o	o	o	o		o	o	o	o	o	o			o	o	o	o	o	
Space/proximity	o										o									o	o	o		o	o				o					o	o		
Listening (basic)	o										o							o		o	o	o		o			o		o			o	o				
Volume, prosody, etc	o										o							o		o				o					o			o	o				
Relaxation																													o								
Touch																									o	o											
Memory	o	o	o								o							o		o				o	o			o	o								
Interaction skills																																					
Greetings											o													o	o								o				
Initiation/asking											o									o							o		o								
Listening (advanced)	o										o									o									o								
Answering/responding											o									o									o								
Topic maintenance																			o	o									o								
Termination	o										o																		o								
Complimenting																																					
Co-operating	o										o							o	o	o	o			o	o	o	o	o	o		o	o	o		o		
Turn-taking, breaking in	o										o							o	o	o	o			o	o	o	o	o	o		o	o	o	o	o		
Affective skills																																					
Identification of feelings																		o	o	o	o					o	o	o	o			o			o		
Recognizing own feelings / other's feelings																		o	o	o	o					o	o	o	o			o		o	o		
Trust	o																	o		o								o				o					
Disclosures										o								o		o								o				o					
Cognitive skills																																					
Social perception																		o		o	o				o		o		o				o		o		
Problem-solving			o																							o	o	o					o		o		
Self-instruction																		o		o						o	o					o				o	
Self-monitoring, etc.	o																	o		o				o					o			o				o	
Negotiating																													o								
Assertion																		o						o					o								

Patient Group: Laryngectomy (contd)

EXERCISE NUMBER:	38	39	40	41	42	43	44	45	46	47	48	49	50	51	52	53	54	55	56	57	58	59	60	61	62	63	64	65	66	67	68	69	70	71	72	73	74
Foundation skills																																					
Gelling																	o	o	o	o							o	o			o	o	o	o	o	o	
Observation			o	o				o	o						o		o	o	o	o						o	o	o		o	o	o	o	o	o	o	
Eye-contact			o	o				o	o						o		o		o	o						o	o	o		o	o	o	o	o	o	o	
Posture			o	o				o	o								o	o												o	o	o	o	o	o	o	
Presentation/grooming															o																	o	o	o	o	o	
Facial expression			o	o				o	o						o		o		o	o						o				o	o	o	o	o	o	o	
Gesture			o	o				o	o								o	o	o							o				o	o	o	o	o	o	o	
Space/proximity			o	o				o	o				o	o			o	o	o				o			o	o			o	o	o		o	o	o	
Listening (basic)			o					o	o				o	o			o	o	o													o		o			
Volume, prosody, etc			o					o	o												o	o										o					
Relaxation																								o													
Touch			o					o							o		o		o		o					o				o	o	o	o	o	o	o	
Memory																																	o	o	o	o	
Interaction skills																																					
Greetings																	o	o	o												o	o			o	o	
Initiation/asking																															o	o	o	o	o		
Listening (advanced)																															o				o		
Answering/responding																																					
Topic maintenance																																					
Termination																															o	o	o	o	o	o	
Complimenting		o						o							o		o	o	o		o					o	o			o	o	o		o	o	o	
Co-operating		o						o									o	o	o		o					o	o			o	o	o		o	o	o	
Turn-taking, breaking in																																					
Affective skills																																					
Identification of feelings	o	o																	o							o				o	o	o	o	o	o	o	
Recognizing own feelings																			o							o				o	o	o	o	o	o	o	
other's feelings		o																	o							o				o	o	o	o	o	o	o	
Trust																			o							o				o	o	o	o	o	o	o	
Disclosures																			o																		
Cognitive skills																																					
Social perception	o	o													o			o	o							o				o	o		o	o	o	o	
Problem-solving	o	o									o				o			o															o				
Self-instruction																										o						o			o	o	
Self-monitoring, etc.																			o							o											
Negotiating																										o						o			o	o	
Assertion																																o			o		o

Patient Group: Laryngectomy (contd)

EXERCISE NUMBER:	75	76	77	78	79	80	81	82	83	84	85	86	87	88	89	90	91	92	93	94	95	96	97	98	99	100	101	102	103	104	105	106	107	108	109	110	111	112	113
Foundation skills																																							
Gelling	o							o											o				o		o	o	o					o	o		o				o
Observation	o							o				o	o						o		o		o		o	o	o				o	o	o		o	o			o
Eye-contact	o							o	o			o	o						o		o	o	o		o	o	o			o	o	o	o		o	o	o		
Posture												o	o					o	o						o	o	o			o	o	o	o						
Presentation/grooming																																							
Facial expression	o							o				o	o				o		o		o	o	o		o	o	o			o	o	o	o		o				
Gesture	o							o				o	o						o			o	o		o	o	o			o	o	o							
Space/proximity	o							o				o	o										o							o	o	o			o	o			
Listening (basic)	o							o				o	o			o			o				o							o	o	o	o		o	o			
Volume, prosody, etc	o							o				o	o						o		o	o	o							o	o	o	o						
Relaxation												o	o									o	o																
Touch	o							o				o	o			o			o																				
Memory	o			o				o				o	o						o			o	o										o		o	o	o		o
Interaction skills																																							
Greetings	o							o				o							o		o	o	o								o	o							
Initiation/asking	o																		o		o	o	o								o	o	o						
Listening (advanced)												o	o					o	o					o							o		o						
Answering/responding								o	o			o												o															
Topic maintenance								o	o			o											o	o															
Termination												o	o																										
Complimenting												o	o						o				o								o	o	o		o	o			o
Co-operating	o							o				o	o				o		o				o								o	o	o			o			o
Turn-taking, breaking in	o							o	o			o	o						o				o									o			o	o			
Affective skills																																							
Identification of feelings	o							o				o							o				o		o	o			o		o		o	o					
Recognizing own feelings	o							o				o							o						o	o			o				o	o					
other's feelings	o											o							o						o	o			o				o	o					
Trust								o				o							o														o						
Disclosures	o							o				o											o										o						
Cognitive skills																																							
Social perception								o				o							o				o				o				o		o						
Problem-solving						o		o				o																					o						
Self-instruction						o		o				o							o			o	o								o		o				o	o	
Self-monitoring, etc.						o		o				o							o			o	o								o		o			o		o	
Negotiating												o																			o		o						
Assertion	o							o				o							o			o	o								o		o						o

Patient Group: Physical Disability

EXERCISE NUMBER:	1	2	3	4	5	6	7	8	9	10	11	12	13	14	15	16	17	18	19	20	21	22	23	24	25	26	27	28	29	30	31	32	33	34	35	36	37
Foundation skills																																					
Gelling		o	o	o	o	o	o	o	o	o	o			o	o		o			o	o			o	o	o	o	o	o				o	o	o	o	o
Observation		o	o	o	o	o	o	o	o	o	o	o	o	o	o	o	o		o	o	o			o	o	o	o	o	o		o	o	o	o	o	o	o
Eye-contact	o	o	o	o	o	o	o	o	o	o	o	o	o	o	o	o	o	o	o	o	o		o	o	o	o	o	o	o		o	o	o	o	o		
Posture	o										o	o	o	o	o	o	o	o	o	o	o			o		o		o	o		o						
Presentation/grooming		o									o	o		o	o		o	o	o	o	o			o	o	o	o	o	o				o	o	o	o	o
Facial expression	o	o			o		o		o		o	o		o	o	o	o	o	o	o	o		o	o	o	o	o	o	o		o		o	o		o	o
Gesture	o				o							o	o	o		o	o			o	o		o	o	o	o		o	o			o	o		o	o	o
Space/proximity	o	o	o				o		o		o			o	o	o	o	o		o			o	o		o	o		o			o	o	o		o	o
Listening (basic)	o	o	o	o		o	o		o								o			o			o			o		o	o								
Volume, prosody, etc	o	o	o	o					o		o			o	o	o	o	o	o	o	o		o	o	o	o	o		o			o					
Relaxation									o	o		o	o													o		o									
Touch	o	o				o					o	o		o	o									o	o	o		o						o			
Memory	o	o	o	o				o			o	o		o		o	o	o		o			o	o	o									o			o
Interaction skills																																					
Greetings					o						o			o	o	o	o		o	o			o	o	o	o	o	o	o				o				
Initiation/asking	o		o	o							o			o	o	o			o	o			o					o	o								
Listening (advanced)	o		o	o							o			o	o	o	o		o	o							o		o								
Answering/responding											o			o	o		o		o	o									o								
Topic maintenance														o			o												o								
Termination	o																																				
Complimenting		o		o	o	o		o			o			o	o	o	o	o	o	o			o	o	o	o	o	o	o		o	o	o	o	o	o	o
Co-operating		o		o	o	o		o			o			o	o	o	o	o	o	o	o		o	o	o	o	o	o	o		o	o	o	o	o	o	o
Turn-taking, breaking in	o	o	o	o	o		o				o		o																								
Affective skills																																					
Identification of feelings				o	o									o	o	o	o	o	o	o						o	o	o	o			o		o	o	o	o
Recognizing own feelings				o	o									o	o	o	o	o	o	o						o	o	o	o			o		o	o	o	o
other's feelings				o	o	o	o										o	o										o	o								
Trust	o										o				o			o						o		o		o	o								
Disclosures																	o	o										o	o								
Cognitive skills																																					
Social perception	o	o	o			o	o							o	o	o	o	o	o	o	o		o	o	o	o	o	o	o		o		o		o	o	o
Problem-solving																							o			o		o	o	o	o	o				o	
Self-instruction	o				o		o																o			o	o	o	o							o	o
Self-monitoring, etc.	o			o	o																		o									o					
Negotiating																								o		o		o	o								
Assertion		o	o																	o									o			o	o		o		o

Patient Group: Physical Disability (contd)

EXERCISE NUMBER:	38	39	40	41	42	43	44	45	46	47	48	49	50	51	52	53	54	55	56	57	58	59	60	61	62	63	64	65	66	67	68	69	70	71	72	73	74
Foundation skills																																					
Gelling	o			o	o	o	o	o	o	o	o	o	o	o	o	o	o	o	o	o				o	o	o	o				o	o	o	o	o	o	o
Observation	o	o		o	o	o	o	o	o	o	o	o	o	o	o	o	o	o	o	o			o	o	o	o	o			o	o	o	o	o	o	o	o
Eye-contact	o	o		o	o				o	o	o	o	o	o	o	o	o	o			o		o	o	o	o	o			o	o	o	o	o	o	o	o
Posture	o	o		o	o				o	o	o	o	o	o		o	o	o	o				o	o	o					o	o	o	o	o	o	o	o
Presentation/grooming																		o												o	o	o					
Facial expression	o	o		o	o				o	o	o	o			o		o	o	o	o			o	o	o	o	o			o	o	o	o	o	o	o	o
Gesture	o	o		o	o				o	o	o	o		o	o	o	o	o	o		o	o	o	o	o	o	o			o	o	o	o	o	o	o	o
Space/proximity			o		o				o	o	o			o	o	o	o	o	o				o	o	o					o	o	o	o	o			
Listening (basic)	o	o		o	o		o	o	o	o	o			o	o	o	o	o	o	o		o	o	o	o	o				o	o	o	o	o	o	o	o
Volume, prosody, etc	o	o		o			o	o	o	o			o		o	o	o	o	o	o		o	o	o	o	o					o	o	o	o	o		o	o
Relaxation													o																								
Touch	o					o	o		o	o	o	o		o	o		o	o			o		o	o	o	o				o	o	o	o	o	o		o
Memory							o	o	o	o	o	o		o	o	o	o		o		o													o		o	
Interaction skills																																					
Greetings	o																														o	o			o	o	o
Initiation/asking	o																				o			o	o						o	o	o	o	o	o	o
Listening (advanced)	o																				o				o						o	o			o	o	
Answering/responding	o								o												o		o								o	o				o	o
Topic maintenance																o															o	o					
Termination																															o	o					
Complimenting																															o	o					
Co-operating	o			o	o	o	o	o	o	o	o	o	o			o	o	o	o		o		o	o	o	o	o			o	o	o	o	o	o		o	o
Turn-taking, breaking in	o			o	o	o	o	o	o	o	o	o		o		o	o	o	o		o		o	o	o	o	o			o	o	o	o	o	o		o	o
Affective skills																																					
Identification of feelings	o		o	o															o					o	o						o	o			o	o	
Recognizing own feelings																			o					o	o						o	o			o	o	
other's feelings			o			o												o	o						o						o	o			o	o	o
Trust																o			o						o						o	o			o	o	
Disclosures																			o						o						o	o			o	o	
Cognitive skills																																					
Social perception	o		o	o											■			o	o					o	o	o	o			o	o	o			o	o	o
Problem-solving	o		o	o						o					■	o		o	o					o	o	o				o	o	o			o	o	o
Self-instruction													o																								
Self-monitoring, etc.																			o					o	o						o	o			o	o	o
Negotiating																o																					o
Assertion	o									o						ɔ																					

Patient Group: Physical Disability (contd)

EXERCISE NUMBER:	75	76	77	78	79	80	81	82	83	84	85	86	87	88	89	90	91	92	93	94	95	96	97	98	99	100	101	102	103	104	105	106	107	108	109	110	111	112	113
Foundation skills																																							
Gelling	o	o	o	o	o	o	o	o	o	o	o	o	o	o		o	o	o	o	o	o	o	o	o	o	o	o		o	o		o	o		o	o			o
Observation	o	o	o	o	o	o	o	o	o	o	o	o	o	o		o	o	o	o	o	o	o	o	o	o	o	o		o	o	o	o	o		o	o	o	o	
Eye-contact	o	o	o	o	o	o	o	o	o	o	o	o	o	o		o	o	o	o	o	o	o	o	o	o	o	o		o	o	o	o	o		o				
Posture	o	o	o	o				o			o	o	o					o			o	o	o	o							o	o	o						
Presentation/grooming	o	o																																					
Facial expression	o	o	o	o		o	o	o	o	o	o	o	o	o	o				o		o	o	o	o	o	o	o	o	o	o	o	o	o		o			o	
Gesture	o	o		o	o			o																															
Space/proximity	o	o	o	o	o	o	o	o	o	o	o	o	o	o		o		o	o	o	o	o	o	o	o	o		o		o	o	o	o		o	o		o	
Listening (basic)	o	o	o	o	o	o	o	o	o	o	o	o	o	o		o		o	o	o	o	o	o	o	o	o					o	o	o						
Volume, prosody, etc	o	o	o	o	o	o	o	o	o		o	o	o	o				o	o	o	o	o	o		o														
Relaxation	o																																						
Touch	o	o	o	o	o	o	o		o	o	o	o		o		o		o	o	o	o	o	o	o	o		o	o	o		o		o			o	o	o	o
Memory	o	o				o																																	
Interaction skills																																							
Greetings	o	o							o	o	o	o	o					o			o	o	o	o							o	o						
Initiation/asking	o	o						o	o	o	o	o	o					o	o		o	o	o					o			o	o	o						
Listening (advanced)												o	o	o					o	o	o	o	o		o					o									
Answering/responding										o	o	o	o																										
Topic maintenance									o	o	o	o	o							o																			
Termination									o	o		o	o							o																			
Complimenting												o	o	o			o	o	o	o			o	o	o	o				o	o	o	o				o	o	
Co-operating	o	o	o	o	o	o	o	o	o	o	o	o	o	o		o	o	o	o	o					o					o									
Turn-taking, breaking in	o	o	o	o	o	o	o	o	o	o	o	o	o	o		o	o	o	o	o	o			o							o		o		o				
Affective skills																																							
Identification of feelings	o	o						o	o	o	o	o	o		o			o	o	o				o		o		o	o	o		o	o	o				o	
Recognizing own feelings	o	o						o	o	o	o	o	o					o	o	o						o		o	o	o		o	o	o					
other's feelings	o	o							o	o	o	o	o					o	o	o						o		o	o	o				o					
Trust	o			o				o	o		o	o	o					o	o	o						o		o	o	o				o					
Disclosures	o								o			o	o											o				o	o	o									
Cognitive skills																																							
Social perception	o					o	o	o	o	o	o	o	o		o		o	o	o					o			o				o	o	o				o		
Problem-solving	o						o	o	o	o	o	o	o					o	o	o			o	o								o	o						
Self-instruction	o	o		o		o		o	o	o	o	o	o		o			o	o	o	o	o	o	o							o		o				o	o	
Self-monitoring, etc.	o	o		o				o	o	o	o	o	o					o	o	o	o	o	o	o								o	o				o	o	o
Negotiating	o								o	o	o	o	o					o	o	o													o						
Assertion	o	o				o		o	o	o	o	o	o			o		o	o	o											o		o						o

Patient Group: Phonological Impairment

EXERCISE NUMBER:	1	2	3	4	5	6	7	8	9	10	11	12	13	14	15	16	17	18	19	20	21	22	23	24	25	26	27	28	29	30	31	32	33	34	35	36	37
Foundation skills																																					
Gelling			o	o	o	o	o	o	o		o			o	o	o	o	o	o	o	o	o	o	o	o	o	o	o	o	o	o	o	o	o	o	o	o
Observation		o	o	o	o	o	o	o	o		o			o	o	o	o	o	o	o	o	o	o	o	o	o	o	o	o	o	o	o	o	o	o	o	o
Eye-contact	o	o	o	o	o	o	o	o	o		o			o	o	o	o	o	o	o	o	o	o	o	o	o	o	o	o	o	o	o	o	o	o	o	o
Posture	o				o	o			o		o			o		o	o			o		o	o	o	o	o	o			o	o			o			
Presentation/grooming																													o								
Facial expression	o			o	o		o				o	o		o	o	o	o	o	o	o	o		o		o	o		o		o		o	o		o		o
Gesture	o			o	o		o				o	o		o	o	o	o	o	o	o	o		o		o	o				o			o		o		o
Space/proximity	o	o		o		o		o	o											o		o					o				o		o				
Listening (basic)	o	o		o	o		o		o	o	o			o	o	o	o	o	o	o	o	o	o		o	o	o	o		o	o	o	o				
Volume, prosody, etc	o			o					o	o	o			o	o					o									o								
Relaxation						o				o																			o								
Touch		o						o																													
Memory	o	o	o	o		o					o	o	o	o		o	o	o	o	o	o	o	o	o	o	o		o	o	o		o	o	o	o	o	o
Interaction skills																																					
Greetings											o			o		o	o		o	o				o	o				o				o			o	o
Initiation/asking	o			o	o						o			o	o					o			o						o							o	o
Listening (advanced)	o			o	o						o			o	o	o	o			o			o				o		o								
Answering/responding											o			o	o	o				o									o								
Topic maintenance														o	o		o			o									o								
Termination	o										o																										
Complimenting																																					
Co-operating				o	o						o			o	o	o	o	o	o	o	o		o		o	o	o	o	o	o	o	o	o	o	o	o	o
Turn-taking, breaking in	o	o		o	o						o	o		o	o	o	o	o	o	o	o		o		o	o	o	o	o	o	o	o	o	o	o	o	o
Affective skills																																					
Identification of feelings				o	o									o	o	o	o	o	o	o					o	o	o	o	o	o	o	o		o	o		
Recognizing own feelings				o	o									o	o	o	o	o	o	o			o		o	o	o	o	o	o	o	o		o	o		
other's feelings				o	o	o								o	o			o	o	o			o					o	o							o	
Trust																	o	o	o									o	o								
Disclosures	o										o			o			o	o							o			o	o								
Cognitive skills																																					
Social perception				o	o		o							o	o	o	o	o	o	o				o		o	o	o	o	o	o	o	o	o	o	o	o
Problem-solving		o	o	o							o			o	o	o	o	o	o	o	o	o	o			o	o	o	o	o	o			o	o	o	
Self-instruction																															o						
Self-monitoring, etc.	o			o	o									o					o	o		o	o	o		o	o				o	o			o	o	o
Negotiating				o	o									o					o				o	o													
Assertion	o	o	o	o										o						o			o	o		o	o	o					o				

Patient Group: Phonological Impairment (contd)

EXERCISE NUMBER:	38	39	40	41	42	43	44	45	46	47	48	49	50	51	52	53	54	55	56	57	58	59	60	61	62	63	64	65	66	67	68	69	70	71	72	73	74
Foundation skills																																					
Gelling				o	o	o			o	o	o	o		o	o		o			o				o	o	o	o	o	o		o	o	o	o	o	o	o
Observation	o	o	o	o	o	o			o	o	o	o		o	o		o			o			o	o	o	o	o	o	o		o	o	o	o	o	o	o
Eye-contact	o		o	o	o	o			o	o	o	o		o	o		o	o		o			o	o	o	o	o	o	o	o	o	o	o		o	o	o
Posture			o		o				o	o	o	o					o	o					o	o	o					o	o	o	o		o	o	
Presentation/grooming	o			o					o	o	o	o					o	o					o	o	o	o		o		o	o	o	o	o	o	o	o
Facial expression		o		o					o	o	o	o	o			o	o	o		o	o		o	o	o	o	o	o	o	o	o	o	o	o	o	o	o
Gesture			o	o	o	o			o	o	o	o	o			o	o	o			o		o	o	o	o		o		o	o	o	o	o	o	o	o
Space/proximity	o	o		o	o				o	o	o	o		o	o		o	o		o			o	o	o	o	o	o	o				o	o	o	o	o
Listening (basic)	o								o	o				o			o	o					o	o	o	o							o	o			
Volume, prosody, etc	o													o									o														
Relaxation																		o			o								o								
Touch			o		o	o			o		o	o	o	o	o	o	o						o	o	o	o	o	o	o	o	o	o	o	o	o	o	o
Memory	o										o														o			o	o	o	o	o	o	o	o	o	o
Interaction skills																																					
Greetings	o								o	o																			o		o	o	o	o	o	o	o
Initiation/asking	o								o	o												o		o					o		o	o	o	o	o	o	o
Listening (advanced)	o								o	o															o						o	o			o	o	
Answering/responding										o	o																				o	o			o	o	
Topic maintenance																															o	o			o	o	
Termination																															o	o			o	o	
Complimenting																								o	o				o	o	o	o	o	o	o	o	o
Co-operating	o			o	o	o			o	o	o	o		o	o	o	o	o		o	o		o	o	o	o	o	o	o	o	o	o	o	o	o	o	o
Turn-taking, breaking in	o			o	o	o			o	o	o	o		o	o	o	o	o		o	o		o	o	o	o	o	o	o	o	o	o	o	o	o	o	o
Affective skills																																					
Identification of feelings	o	o																						o	o	o	o	o	o	o	o	o	o	o	o	o	
Recognizing own feelings																								o	o	o	o	o	o	o	o	o	o	o	o	o	
other's feelings				o																																	
Trust						o																	o		o						o	o			o	o	
Disclosures																		o		o											o	o			o	o	
Cognitive skills																																					
Social perception	o			o	o										o	o	o	o		o					o	o		o	o		o	o	o		o	o	o
Problem-solving				o	o								o		o	o									o		o					o			o	o	
Self-instruction										o																					o						
Self-monitoring, etc.									o																o												
Negotiating						o										o		o					o			o						o			o	o	o
Assertion									o																							o			o	o	

Patient Group: Phonological Impairment (contd)

EXERCISE NUMBER:	75	76	77	78	79	80	81	82	83	84	85	86	87	88	89	90	91	92	93	94	95	96	97	98	99	100	101	102	103	104	105	106	107	108	109	110	111	112	113
Foundation skills																																							
Gelling	o	o	o	o	o	o	o	o	o	o	o	o	o	o	o			o	o	o	o		o	o	o	o	o	o	o	o	o	o	o	o	o	o	o	o	o
Observation	o	o	o	o	o	o	o	o	o	o	o	o	o	o	o	o	o	o	o				o	o	o	o	o	o	o	o	o	o	o	o	o	o	o	o	
Eye-contact	o	o	o	o	o			o	o	o	o	o	o	o	o	o	o	o	o				o		o		o	o	o	o	o	o	o	o	o	o			
Posture	o	o			o	o					o		o	o	o	o				o								o		o	o	o							
Presentation/grooming	o																																						
Facial expression	o	o		o	o			o	o	o	o	o	o	o	o			o	o	o			o	o	o	o	o	o	o	o	o	o	o	o	o				
Gesture	o	o		o				o	o	o	o	o	o	o	o	o		o	o	o			o		o	o	o	o		o	o	o	o	o	o				
Space/proximity	o	o	o			o	o	o	o	o	o	o	o	o				o	o	o									o	o	o	o	o	o	o	o	o		
Listening (basic)	o	o	o			o	o	o	o	o	o	o	o	o	o	o		o	o	o			o	o	o	o	o			o	o	o	o	o		o		o	o
Volume, prosody, etc	o	o	o			o	o	o	o	o	o	o	o	o	o		o		o	o			o	o						o	o	o	o	o	o	o	o	o	o
Relaxation	o																																						
Touch	o	o	o	o			o	o	o	o	o	o	o	o	o	o		o	o	o			o	o	o		o	o					o						
Memory	o	o					o	o	o	o	o	o	o	o	o			o	o	o			o	o	o														o
Interaction skills																																							
Greetings	o	o							o	o	o	o	o	o				o	o											o	o	o	o	o					
Initiation/asking	o	o						o	o	o	o	o	o				o	o	o		o	o	o							o	o	o	o	o					o
Listening (advanced)								o	o	o	o	o	o	o				o	o				o							o	o	o							
Answering/responding								o	o	o	o	o	o											o															
Topic maintenance								o		o	o	o	o										o																
Termination									o		o	o	o						o																				
Complimenting				o	o						o	o	o	o				o	o											o	o	o	o	o				o	o
Co-operating	o	o		o	o		o	o		o	o	o	o	o	o	o		o	o	o			o	o						o	o	o	o	o		o			
Turn-taking, breaking in	o	o		o	o		o	o	o	o	o	o	o	o	o	o		o	o	o														o					
Affective skills																																							
Identification of feelings								o	o		o	o	o	o				o	o	o			o	o		o	o	o		o	o	o		o					
Recognizing own feelings	o	o						o			o	o	o	o				o	o	o			o	o		o	o	o		o	o	o		o				o	o
other's feelings	o	o						o			o	o	o	o				o	o	o						o	o	o		o	o							o	o
Trust	o				o			o	o		o	o			o			o	o	o				o		o	o	o											
Disclosures	o				o			o	o		o	o						o	o	o				o		o	o	o					o						
Cognitive skills																																							
Social perception	o							o	o		o	o	o	o		o		o	o															o					
Problem-solving								o	o		o	o	o	o		o			o																				
Self-instruction	o	o			o	o		o	o		o	o	o	o		o		o	o	o			o	o			o			o	o	o	o					o	o
Self-monitoring, etc.	o				o	o		o	o		o	o	o	o		o			o	o			o	o						o	o	o					o	o	
Negotiating								o	o		o	o	o	o					o	o										o	o	o							
Assertion	o							o	o		o	o	o	o		o		o	o	o			o	o						o	o	o							o

Patient Group: Mental Illness

EXERCISE NUMBER:	1	2	3	4	5	6	7	8	9	10	11	12	13	14	15	16	17	18	19	20	21	22	23	24	25	26	27	28	29	30	31	32	33	34	35	36	37
Foundation skills																																					
Gelling		o	o	o	o			o		o		o		o	o	o	o						o	o	o	o	o	o	o			o	o	o	o		o
Observation	o	o	o	o	o	o		o			o	o		o	o	o	o		o	o	o		o	o	o	o	o	o	o				o	o	o	o	o
Eye-contact	o	o	o	o	o	o		o			o	o		o	o		o		o	o			o	o	o	o	o	o	o			o	o	o		o	o
Posture	o							o				o	o	o	o	o	o			o	o			o													
Presentation/grooming	o									o	o	o		o	o	o	o	o	o	o	o			o	o	o	o		o			o	o	o		o	o
Facial expression	o			o						o	o	o		o	o	o	o	o		o	o		o	o	o	o	o		o			o	o	o		o	o
Gesture	o		o	o	o		o			o	o			o	o	o	o			o	o		o	o	o				o				o	o		o	o
Space/proximity	o	o								o	o			o	o	o	o			o	o		o	o			o	o	o			o	o		o	o	o
Listening (basic)	o	o								o	o				o	o	o	o	o	o	o		o	o					o								o
Volume, prosody, etc	o									o				o									o	o													
Relaxation											o		o												o	o		o									
Touch	o	o						o			o	o			o									o													
Memory	o	o	o							o	o					o	o	o	o	o			o	o		o		o	o								o
Interaction skills																																					
Greetings					o						o			o	o	o	o			o			o	o	o				o				o		o		o
Initiation/asking			o		o						o				o	o	o		o	o			o				o		o								o
Listening (advanced)	o		o		o						o				o	o			o	o									o								o
Answering/responding														o	o					o									o								o
Topic maintenance	o										o				o					o									o								o
Termination	o														o														o								
Complimenting	o										o	o		o	o	o	o	o	o	o			o	o	o	o	o	o	o			o	o	o	o	o	o
Co-operating	o	o		o	o						o			o	o	o	o	o	o	o			o	o	o	o	o	o	o			o	o	o	o	o	o
Turn-taking, breaking in	o	o			o						o	o																									
Affective skills																																					
Identification of feelings				o											o	o	o	o	o	o	o					o	o	o	o								
Recognizing own feelings				o											o	o	o	o	o	o						o	o	o	o								
other's feelings				o													o	o										o	o								
Trust																		o	o							o	o										
Disclosures	o							o			o				o			o		o				o													
Cognitive skills																																					
Social perception														o	o	o	o	o		o	o				o	o	o	o	o			o	o		o	o	o
Problem-solving		o	o								o					o	o						o			o	o										
Self-instruction																	o						o			o	o					o				o	
Self-monitoring, etc.	o			o	o													o		o			o	o		o		o	o			o					
Negotiating																							o			o		o	o								
Assertion		o													o									o													

Patient Group: Mental Illness (contd)

EXERCISE NUMBER:	38	39	40	41	42	43	44	45	46	47	48	49	50	51	52	53	54	55	56	57	58	59	60	61	62	63	64	65	66	67	68	69	70	71	72	73	74
Foundation skills																																					
Gelling																	o	o		o				o	o	o	o	o	o	o	o	o	o	o	o	o	
Observation0	o	o					o	o	o	o	o			o	o		o	o		o	o	o	o	o	o	o	o	o	o	o	o	o	o	o	o	o	o
Eye-contact	o	o					o	o	o	o	o			o	o		o	o		o	o	o	o	o	o	o	o	o	o	o	o	o	o	o	o	o	o
Posture								o	o				o		o		o							o	o		o	o	o		o	o	o			o	
Presentation/grooming																																					
Facial expression	o		o				o	o	o					o			o			o			o	o	o	o					o	o	o		o		o
Gesture	o	o					o	o	o														o	o	o				o		o	o					
Space/proximity	o	o		o			o	o	o				o	o			o	o	o	o			o	o	o		o		o		o	o	o				
Listening (basic)	o						o	o	o				o	o			o	o		o			o	o	o						o	o		o		o	o
Volume, prosody, etc	o						o	o	o				o	o						o			o	o	o						o	o	o	o			
Relaxation																																					
Touch	o			o			o		o		o			o	o		o		o	o			o	o	o	o		o	o	o	o	o	o	o	o	o	o
Memory	o			o			o	o			o			o	o													o	o		o					o	
Interaction skills																																					
Greetings	o																				o	o			o						o	o	o	o	o	o	
Initiation/asking	o																	o			o	o		o							o	o	o	o	o	o	
Listening (advanced)	o																	o			o	o			o												
Answering/responding									o														o														
Topic maintenance																							o														
Termination																																					
Complimenting																															o	o					
Co-operating	o			o			o	o	o		o			o			o	o	o	o			o	o	o	o		o	o	o	o	o	o		o	o	
Turn-taking, breaking in	o			o			o	o	o		o		o				o	o	o	o			o	o	o	o		o	o	o	o	o	o		o	o	
Affective skills																																					
Identification of feelings	o	o																	o					o	o	o	o	o	o	o	o	o	o	o	o	o	
Recognizing own feelings																			o					o	o	o	o	o	o	o	o	o	o	o	o	o	
other's feelings			o																o						o	o	o	o	o	o	o	o	o	o	o		o	
Trust						o													o					o	o	o	o	o	o	o	o	o					
Disclosures																			o			o															
Cognitive skills																																					
Social perception	o	o												o	o		o	o	o					o	o	o		o		o	o	o	o		o	o	
Problem-solving	o	o											o	o	o		o	o	o					o	o	o		o		o	o	o	o		o	o	
Self-instruction									o										o												o				o		o
Self-monitoring, etc.							o												o												o						
Negotiating																																					
Assertion							o																								o				o		o

Patient Group: Mental Illness (contd)

EXERCISE NUMBER:	75	76	77	78	79	80	81	82	83	84	85	86	87	88	89	90	91	92	93	94	95	96	97	98	99	100	101	102	103	104	105	106	107	108	109	110	111	112	113
Foundation skills																																							
Gelling				o	o		o	o	o	o				o	o			o	o	o			o	o	o	o	o	o	o	o		o	o	o		o	o	o	
Observation	o		o	o	o		o	o	o				o	o	o		o	o	o	o		o	o	o	o	o	o	o		o	o	o	o	o		o	o	o	
Eye-contact		o					o	o	o			o	o	o	o	o	o		o			o	o	o	o	o	o	o		o	o	o	o		o		o		
Posture							o		o	o		o							o	o				o	o	o	o	o											
Presentation/grooming	o						o		o	o	o	o	o	o	o			o	o				o	o	o	o	o	o	o	o	o	o	o	o					
Facial expression	o						o		o	o	o	o	o	o	o			o	o			o	o	o		o	o	o	o	o	o	o	o						
Gesture	o	o			o		o		o	o		o	o	o	o			o	o			o	o	o					o	o	o	o							
Space/proximity	o	o					o		o	o	o	o	o	o	o		o	o	o	o			o	o	o	o	o	o	o	o	o	o	o	o		o	o	o	
Listening (basic)	o	o							o	o	o	o	o	o	o		o	o	o	o	o	o	o	o	o	o	o	o	o	o	o	o				o	o	o	
Volume, prosody, etc	o	o							o	o			o										o																
Relaxation	o																																						
Touch	o	o		o	o		o		o	o	o	o	o				o	o	o	o	o	o	o	o	o	o	o	o	o	o		o	o						
Memory	o	o					o		o	o	o																o												
Interaction skills																																							
Greetings	o	o							o	o		o	o	o				o	o	o	o	o	o	o							o	o	o	o					
Initiation/asking	o	o							o	o		o	o	o				o	o	o	o	o	o	o							o	o	o						
Listening (advanced)												o	o					o	o	o	o										o	o							
Answering/responding									o	o		o	o	o				o	o	o		o	o								o	o							
Topic maintenance									o	o		o	o	o				o	o	o		o	o		o						o	o							
Termination												o	o	o			o	o	o												o	o							
Complimenting	o	o					o	o	o	o	o	o	o	o	o		o	o	o	o	o		o	o							o	o		o					o
Co-operating	o	o					o	o	o	o	o	o	o	o	o		o	o	o	o	o									o	o	o							
Turn-taking, breaking in														o						o																			
Affective skills																																							
Identification of feelings	o	o							o	o		o	o	o	o			o	o	o	o			o		o	o	o			o	o	o	o					
Recognizing own feelings	o	o							o	o		o	o	o	o			o	o	o	o			o		o	o	o				o	o	o					
other's feelings	o	o																o	o	o	o			o		o	o	o											
Trust	o								o	o		o	o	o	o			o	o	o	o			o		o	o	o											
Disclosures									o	o		o	o			o																							
Cognitive skills																																							
Social perception									o	o		o	o	o	o			o	o		o		o	o							o	o							
Problem-solving									o	o		o	o	o				o	o	o		o	o			o					o	o							
Self-instruction							o	o	o	o		o	o	o				o	o	o		o	o								o	o				o	o		
Self-monitoring, etc.							o	o	o	o		o	o	o						o		o	o	o							o	o					o		
Negotiating									o	o		o	o				o			o											o	o							
Assertion	o						o	o	o	o		o	o	o				o	o	o		o	o	o							o	o							o

Patient Group: Hearing Impairment

EXERCISE NUMBER:	1	2	3	4	5	6	7	8	9	10	11	12	13	14	15	16	17	18	19	20	21	22	23	24	25	26	27	28	29	30	31	32	33	34	35	36	37
Foundation skills																																					
Gelling		o	o	o	o	o	o	o			o			o	o	o	o		o	o			o	o	o	o		o	o	o	o	o	o	o	o		o
Observation		o	o	o	o	o	o	o	o				o	o	o	o	o		o	o	o	o	o	o	o	o	o	o	o	o	o	o	o	o	o	o	o
Eye-contact	o	o	o	o	o	o	o	o	o		o			o	o	o	o	o	o	o	o	o	o	o	o	o	o	o	o	o	o	o	o	o	o	o	o
Posture	o			o	o	o	o	o	o		o			o	o			o	o	o			o	o	o	o			o		o		o	o			
Presentation/grooming																													o								
Facial expression	o				o			o			o	o	o	o	o	o	o	o	o	o	o		o	o	o	o	o	o	o	o	o		o	o	o	o	o
Gesture	o				o		o	o	o		o	o		o	o	o	o	o	o	o	o	o	o	o	o	o	o	o	o	o	o	o	o	o	o	o	o
Space/proximity	o	o	o								o				o		o			o				o			o		o			o	o				o
Listening (basic)	o	o	o	o	o		o		o		o			o	o	o	o	o	o	o	o	o		o	o	o			o	o		o	o	o	o	o	o
Volume, prosody, etc	o			o	o				o		o			o					o	o				o					o			o			o	o	o
Relaxation						o			o				o													o		o		o							
Touch	o	o									o	o			o							o							o								
Memory	o	o	o	o				o			o	o	o	o	o	o	o	o	o		o	o	o	o	o		o	o	o	o				o			
Interaction skills																																						
Greetings		o									o			o	o	o	o		o	o			o	o	o			o	o			o	o		o	o	o
Initiation/asking	o			o	o						o				o	o			o				o				o	o								o	o
Listening (advanced)	o				o						o				o	o	o		o				o					o								o	o
Answering/responding					o						o				o				o									o								o	o
Topic maintenance	o														o		o		o								o		o							o	o
Termination	o														o		o		o										o							o	
Complimenting																													o	o	o						
Co-operating	o	o	o	o	o		o	o	o		o		o	o	o	o	o	o	o		o		o	o	o	o	o	o	o	o	o	o	o	o	o	o	o
Turn-taking, breaking in	o	o	o	o	o						o		o	o	o	o	o	o	o	o	o	o	o	o	o	o	o	o	o	o	o	o	o	o	o	o	o
Affective skills																																						
Identification of feelings				o	o										o		o	o	o	o				o	o	o	o	o	o	o		o					o
Recognizing own feelings				o	o										o			o	o						o	o	o	o	o	o		o		o	o		o
other's feelings				o	o	o	o								o		o	o	o						o	o		o	o	o		o		o	o		o
Trust																		o					o					o				o					o
Disclosures	o									o								o					o		o			o				o					
Cognitive skills																																						
Social perception													o		o	o	o	o	o	o	o		o		o	o	o	o	o	o	o	o	o		o	o	o
Problem-solving						o									o	o	o	o	o				o	o		o	o		o	o				o			
Self-instruction			o																				o	o	o												
Self-monitoring, etc.	o														o		o	o	o	o	o	o	o	o	o			o				o			o		o
Negotiating																																o					
Assertion				o											o																						

Patient Group: Hearing Impairment (contd)

EXERCISE NUMBER:	38	39	40	41	42	43	44	45	46	47	48	49	50	51	52	53	54	55	56	57	58	59	60	61	62	63	64	65	66	67	68	69	70	71	72	73	74
Foundation skills																																					
Gelling	o		o	o	o	o	o	o	o	o	o	o		o	o	o	o		o	o		o	o	o	o	o	o	o	o	o	o	o	o	o	o	o	o
Observation	o	o	o	o	o	o	o	o	o	o	o	o		o	o	o	o	o	o	o	o	o	o	o	o	o	o	o	o	o	o	o	o	o	o	o	o
Eye-contact		o	o	o	o	o	o		o	o	o	o		o	o		o				o	o	o	o	o	o		o		o	o	o	o	o	o	o	
Posture	o	o	o		o			o	o			o	o	o	o		o		o									o	o		o	o	o	o	o	o	o
Presentation/grooming	o																													o							
Facial expression	o		o	o	o	o	o	o	o	o	o	o		o	o	o	o	o		o	o				o	o		o	o	o	o	o	o	o	o	o	o
Gesture			o	o	o	o	o	o	o	o	o	o	o	o	o	o	o	o	o	o	o	o	o	o	o	o	o	o	o		o	o	o				
Space/proximity	o	o	o																								o		o		o						
Listening (basic)	o	o		o					o	o	o	o		o	o	o	o	o	o	o	o	o	o	o	o	o					o	o	o	o	o	o	o
Volume, prosody, etc	o						o	o	o	o	o	o	o			o	o	o	o	o	o	o	o	o	o	o					o	o	o	o	o	o	o
Relaxation	o																																				
Touch			o	o	o	o		o	o	o						o			o	o						o	o	o	o					o			
Memory	o				o	o			o	o	o	o	o	o	o	o	o	o	o	o	o	o	o	o	o	o			o	o	o	o	o	o	o	o	o
Interaction skills																																					
Greetings	o																		o	o	o							o	o	o	o	o	o	o		o	o
Initiation/asking	o																		o	o	o	o	o	o	o	o	o	o	o	o	o	o	o	o	o	o	o
Listening (advanced)	o																		o		o			o	o			o			o	o			o		
Answering/responding									o																												
Topic maintenance																																					
Termination																																					
Complimenting	o		o	o	o	o	o	o	o	o	o	o		o	o	o	o	o	o	o	o	o	o	o	o	o	o	o	o	o	o	o	o	o	o	o	o
Co-operating	o		o	o	o	o	o	o	o	o	o	o		o	o	o	o	o	o	o	o	o	o	o	o	o	o	o	o	o	o	o	o	o	o	o	o
Turn-taking, breaking in	o																																				
Affective skills																																					
Identification of feelings		o	o												o	o	o		o			o	o	o	o	o	o	o	o	o	o	o	o	o	o	o		
Recognizing own feelings																			o			o	o	o	o	o	o	o	o	o	o	o					
other's feelings				o															o								o		o	o	o	o					
Trust				o															o						o												
Disclosures																					o								o	o	o						
Cognitive skills																																					
Social perception	o		o	o									o		o	o	o	o	o			o	o	o	o	o	o	o	o	o	o	o	o	o	o	o	o
Problem-solving			o	o												o					o		o		o	o		o			o		o	o	o		o
Self-instruction									o																												
Self-monitoring, etc.																o		o									o					o					
Negotiating					o																				o												o
Assertion										o																											

Patient Group: Hearing Impairment (contd)

EXERCISE NUMBER:	75	76	77	78	79	80	81	82	83	84	85	86	87	88	89	90	91	92	93	94	95	96	97	98	99	100	101	102	103	104	105	106	107	108	109	110	111	112	113
Foundation skills																																							
Gelling	o	o	o	o	o	o	o	o	o	o			o			o			o				o	o	o	o	o	o	o	o	o	o	o	o	o	o	o	o	o
Observation	o	o	o	o	o	o	o	o	o	o	o	o	o	o		o			o				o	o	o	o	o	o	o	o	o	o	o	o	o	o	o	o	o
Eye-contact	o	o	o	o	o	o			o	o	o	o	o	o	o	o	o		o				o	o	o	o		o		o	o	o	o	o		o	o	o	o
Posture	o	o			o	o				o	o	o	o	o	o	o		o	o	o			o	o	o	o		o	o	o	o	o	o						
Presentation/grooming	o	o			o	o							o																										
Facial expression	o	o			o	o			o	o	o	o	o	o	o	o	o		o		o		o	o	o	o		o	o	o	o	o	o	o		o			
Gesture	o	o			o	o			o	o	o	o	o	o	o	o	o		o				o	o	o	o		o	o	o	o	o	o	o					
Space/proximity	o	o			o	o	o	o	o	o	o	o	o	o	o				o				o	o				o	o	o	o	o							
Listening (basic)	o	o		o	o	o	o	o	o	o	o	o	o	o	o	o			o				o		o	o		o	o	o	o	o		o		o	o	o	o
Volume, prosody, etc	o	o		o	o	o			o	o	o	o	o	o	o	o			o				o	o				o	o	o	o	o	o		o	o	o	o	o
Relaxation	o																		o																				
Touch	o	o	o	o					o	o	o	o				o			o				o			o		o	o										
Memory	o	o	o	o			o		o	o	o	o	o	o		o	o		o				o		o	o		o	o	o	o	o	o	o		o	o	o	o
Interaction skills																																							
Greetings	o	o									o										o																		
Initiation/asking	o	o							o	o	o	o									o	o	o							o	o	o		o	o				o
Listening (advanced)											o	o		o		o							o							o	o	o							
Answering/responding											o	o											o							o	o	o							
Topic maintenance									o	o	o	o										o		o															
Termination									o	o	o	o										o		o															
Complimenting	o	o	o	o	o	o			o	o	o	o	o	o		o	o		o				o		o	o		o	o	o	o	o	o		o	o	o	o	o
Co-operating	o	o	o	o	o	o	o	o	o	o	o	o	o	o		o	o		o				o	o	o	o		o	o	o	o	o	o		o				o
Turn-taking, breaking in						o					o	o				o			o				o							o			o		o				
Affective skills																																							
Identification of feelings	o					o			o	o	o	o	o			o			o				o		o	o	o	o		o		o							
Recognizing own feelings	o					o			o	o	o	o	o						o				o		o	o	o	o				o							
other's feelings	o					o					o	o	o						o				o		o	o	o	o				o							
Trust	o				o				o	o	o	o	o		o				o				o		o	o	o	o											
Disclosures	o				o				o	o	o	o	o	o					o				o		o	o	o	o		o									
Cognitive skills																																							
Social perception	o					o			o	o	o	o	o		o				o				o		o	o				o									
Problem-solving						o			o	o	o	o	o		o	o			o				o				o	o											
Self-instruction	o	o				o			o	o	o	o	o			o			o				o		o	o				o	o	o		o		o	o	o	
Self-monitoring, etc.	o	o				o			o	o	o	o	o		o				o				o		o	o				o	o	o		o		o	o	o	o
Negotiating										o	o	o	o			o			o													o							
Assertion	o					o			o	o	o	o	o						o				o		o	o				o									o

Patient Group: Stutter

EXERCISE NUMBER:	1	2	3	4	5	6	7	8	9	10	11	12	13	14	15	16	17	18	19	20	21	22	23	24	25	26	27	28	29	30	31	32	33	34	35	36	37
Foundation skills																																					
Gelling	o	o	o	o	o	o	o	o	o	o	o			o	o	o	o			o	o		o	o	o	o	o	o	o	o	o	o	o	o	o	o	o
Observation	o	o	o	o	o	o	o	o	o	o	o	o		o	o	o	o		o	o	o		o	o	o	o	o	o	o	o	o	o	o	o		o	o
Eye-contact	o	o	o	o	o	o	o	o	o	o	o		o	o		o	o		o	o			o	o	o	o	o	o	o	o	o	o	o	o	o		o
Posture	o			o	o	o	o	o	o	o		o	o																								
Presentation/grooming							o	o					o																o								
Facial expression	o	o			o	o			o	o	o	o		o	o	o	o	o		o	o		o	o	o	o		o	o					o	o	o	o
Gesture	o	o			o	o	o	o	o	o	o	o		o	o	o	o	o	o	o	o		o	o	o	o	o	o	o		o	o	o	o	o	o	o
Space/proximity	o	o	o	o		o		o	o	o	o			o	o	o	o	o		o	o		o	o		o	o	o	o			o		o			o
Listening (basic)	o	o	o	o		o		o	o	o	o			o	o	o	o	o	o	o	o		o	o	o	o	o	o	o	o	o	o	o	o	o	o	o
Volume, prosody, etc	o	o		o		o			o	o	o			o	o	o	o	o		o	o		o	o		o	o	o	o		o	o	o	o	o	o	o
Relaxation						o			o	o		o	o		o														o	o							
Touch	o	o				o		o			o	o			o		o					o	o	o	o	o		o	o								
Memory	o	o	o								o	o	o		o		o	o				o	o	o	o	o		o						o			o
Interaction skills																																					
Greetings					o						o		o	o	o	o	o			o			o		o				o				o				o
Initiation/asking	o				o						o			o	o	o	o	o		o			o			o		o	o						o		o
Listening (advanced)	o				o	o					o				o	o		o		o			o				o		o						o		o
Answering/responding											o				o		o	o		o			o	o	o			o	o	o							o
Topic maintenance	o												o	o	o	o	o			o			o	o	o			o	o								
Termination	o										o		o	o	o					o								o	o		o						
Complimenting											o				o	o	o	o	o	o			o	o			o	o	o	o	o	o	o	o	o	o	o
Co-operating	o	o			o						o			o	o	o	o	o	o	o		o	o	o	o		o	o	o	o	o	o	o	o	o	o	o
Turn-taking, breaking in	o	o			o						o	o	o	o	o	o	o	o	o	o			o	o	o			o	o	o	o	o	o	o	o	o	o
Affective skills																																					
Identification of feelings															o		o	o	o	o	o							o	o	o	o	o		o	o		
Recognizing own feelings																o	o	o	o	o						o	o	o	o	o	o	o		o	o	o	
other's feelings							o								o		o			o			o					o	o	o		o			o		o
Trust																	o	o								o	o										
Disclosures	o										o				o	o	o	o			o		o					o	o								
Cognitive skills																																					
Social perception											o			o	o	o	o	o		o	o		o	o	o	o	o	o	o	o	o		o		o		o
Problem-solving	o	o	o			o						o								o		o	o			o	o	o	o		o			o		o	
Self-instruction	o																o	o					o									o			o		o
Self-monitoring, etc.																	o	o					o	o		o		o	o								
Negotiating																												o				o					
Assertion	o	o																																			

Patient Group: Stutter (contd)

EXERCISE NUMBER:	38	39	40	41	42	43	44	45	46	47	48	49	50	51	52	53	54	55	56	57	58	59	60	61	62	63	64	65	66	67	68	69	70	71	72	73	74
Foundation skills																																					
Gelling			○	○	○	○	○	○		○	○	○	○	○		○	○	○	○	○			○	○	○	○	○	○			○	○	○	○	○	○	○
Observation	○	○	○	○	○	○	○	○	○	○	○	○	○	○	○	○	○	○	○	○			○	○	○	○	○	○	○	○	○	○	○	○	○	○	○
Eye-contact	○		○	○						○	○	○		○	○	○	○	○	○	○			○	○	○	○	○	○	○	○	○	○	○	○	○	○	○
Posture	○	○	○	○	○					○	○	○	○		○		○	○		○			○				○	○	○	○	○	○	○	○	○	○	○
Presentation/grooming													○																								
Facial expression	○		○	○			○	○	○	○	○	○		○	○	○	○	○		○	○	○	○	○	○	○	○	○	○	○	○	○	○	○	○		
Gesture			○	○			○	○	○	○	○	○		○	○	○	○	○			○	○	○	○	○	○		○		○	○	○	○	○	○	○	○
Space/proximity	○	○			○	○							○				○			○							○		○								
Listening (basic)	○	○	○	○			○	○	○	○	○	○	○		○	○	○	○	○		○	○	○	○	○	○		○	○	○	○	○	○	○	○	○	○
Volume, prosody, etc	○	○					○	○					●	○	○	○	○	○	○		○	○	○	○	○	○		○	○	○	○				○	○	
Relaxation		○											●																								
Touch																												○	○								
Memory	○		○	○	○		○	○		○	○	○	○	○		○	○	○			○	○	○		○	○	○	○	○	○	○	○			○		○
Interaction skills																																					
Greetings	○																														○	○			○		○
Initiation/asking	○																			○	○		○	○							○	○	○	○	○	○	○
Listening (advanced)	○																			○				○							○	○			○	○	
Answering/responding									○																○						○	○			○		○
Topic maintenance																															○	○			○		○
Termination																							○								○	○			○		○
Complimenting																																					
Co-operating	○				○	○	○	○	○	○	○	○				○	○	○		○	○	○	○	○	○	○	○	○	○	○	○	○	○	○	○	○	○
Turn-taking, breaking in	○					○	○	○	○	○	○	○	○	○	○	○	○	○			○	○	○	○	○	○	○	○	○	○	○	○	○	○	○	○	○
Affective skills																																					
Identification of feelings		○	○												○	○		○	○									○	○	○	○	○			○		
Recognizing own feelings			○												○	○		○	○									○	○	○	○	○			○		
other's feelings					○														○									○	○	○	○	○			○		
Trust																			○					○				○	○	○	○						
Disclosures																			○					○	○	○		○	○	○	○						
Cognitive skills																																					
Social perception	○		○	○										○	○		○	○			○			○	○	○		○	○	○	○	○	○	○	○	○	○
Problem-solving			○	○										○	○		○	○			○			○	○	○		○	○	○	○	○	○	○	○	○	○
Self-instruction							○																○								○	○			○		
Self-monitoring, etc.																	○						○								○	○			○	○	
Negotiating						○						○				○															○	○					
Assertion	○																		○							○		○	○	○	○	○			○		○

Patient Group: Stutter (contd)

EXERCISE NUMBER:	75	76	77	78	79	80	81	82	83	84	85	86	87	88	89	90	91	92	93	94	95	96	97	98	99	100	101	102	103	104	105	106	107	108	109	110	111	112	113
Foundation skills																																							
Gelling	o	o	o	o	o	o	o	o	o						o	o	o	o	o	o	o	o	o	o	o	o	o	o	o	o		o	o	o	o	o	o	o	o
Observation	o	o	o	o	o	o	o	o	o						o	o	o	o	o	o	o	o	o	o	o	o	o	o	o		o	o	o	o	o	o	o	o	o
Eye-contact	o	o	o	o	o	o	o		o			o	o	o	o	o	o	o	o	o	o	o	o	o	o	o	o	o	o	o	o		o	o	o				
Posture	o		o			o	o		o			o	o	o	o		o			o			o		o			o							o				o
Presentation/grooming	o						o		o			o	o	o	o				o	o	o	o	o		o	o	o	o	o	o	o	o	o	o					
Facial expression	o	o		o			o		o	o		o	o	o	o	o		o	o	o	o	o	o	o	o	o	o	o	o	o	o	o	o	o	o				o
Gesture	o	o	o		o		o		o		o	o	o	o		o		o	o	o					o		o			o	o	o	o	o	o				
Space/proximity	o	o		o		o	o		o			o		o				o	o	o	o	o	o	o	o	o	o	o	o	o	o	o	o			o	o		o
Listening (basic)	o	o	o		o		o		o			o					o			o	o	o	o	o						o	o	o							
Volume, prosody, etc	o						o		o			o								o	o	o	o	o	o								o						o
Relaxation	o																									o													
Touch	o	o	o	o		o		o	o	o	o	o				o		o	o		o		o	o	o	o			o				o						o
Memory		o	o	o			o	o	o	o								o		o							o												
Interaction skills																																							
Greetings	o	o									o	o									o	o	o	o						o	o	o	o	o					
Initiation/asking	o	o					o		o		o	o					o	o			o	o								o	o	o	o	o					
Listening (advanced)												o		o			o	o				o	o	o															
Answering/responding							o	o			o	o																											
Topic maintenance									o	o		o				o	o	o	o	o	o	o																	
Termination												o	o																										
Complimenting	o	o	o	o			o	o	o	o	o	o	o	o	o		o	o	o	o													o	o					
Co-operating	o	o	o	o			o		o	o	o	o	o	o		o	o	o	o	o										o	o	o	o	o	o				
Turn-taking, breaking in	o	o	o	o			o		o	o	o	o	o	o			o	o	o	o		o	o	o											o				
Affective skills																																							
Identification of feelings	o								o	o	o	o	o	o				o		o	o					o	o	o	o	o	o	o	o	o					
Recognizing own feelings	o								o			o	o	o				o		o	o					o	o	o	o	o	o	o	o						
other's feelings	o											o		o				o		o						o	o	o	o				o							
Trust	o							o			o	o		o				o	o				o			o	o	o	o				o							
Disclosures	o							o			o	o												o		o	o	o	o											
Cognitive skills																																							
Social perception	o					o	o		o	o	o	o	o	o	o			o	o	o			o	o		o					o					o			
Problem-solving							o		o	o	o	o	o	o	o		o	o	o																				
Self-instruction	o	o			o		o		o	o	o	o	o					o	o		o	o	o	o						o	o	o					o	o	
Self-monitoring, etc.	o	o					o		o	o	o	o	o			o		o	o		o	o	o	o							o	o							o
Negotiating							o		o			o	o		o			o	o																				
Assertion	o						o		o			o	o																										

Patient Group: Dysphasia

EXERCISE NUMBER:	1	2	3	4	5	6	7	8	9	10	11	12	13	14	15	16	17	18	19	20	21	22	23	24	25	26	27	28	29	30	31	32	33	34	35	36	37
Foundation skills																																					
Gelling		o	o		o						o		o	o						o				o	o	o	o		o			o	o			o	o
Observation		o	o		o						o	o	o	o	o	o				o	o			o	o	o	o		o			o	o		o	o	o
Eye-contact	o	o	o	o	o					o	o	o	o	o	o	o				o				o	o	o	o		o				o		o	o	o
Posture	o			o	o					o	o	o	o	o	o					o		o		o		o	o		o								
Presentation/grooming													o			o																					
Facial expression	o			o	o						o	o	o	o	o		o	o		o	o			o	o	o	o		o			o	o		o	o	o
Gesture	o			o	o						o	o	o	o	o	o	o	o		o				o	o				o		o	o	o		o	o	o
Space/proximity	o	o	o								o	o		o	o					o				o			o		o			o	o			o	o
Listening (basic)	o	o									o	o		o	o	o	o	o		o				o	o	o	o		o			o	o		o	o	o
Volume, prosody, etc	o										o			o	o					o							o		o								
Relaxation													o																								
Touch	o											o	o											o		o			o								
Memory	o	o	o								o	o	o	o		o		o		o				o	o				o								o
Interaction skills																																					
Greetings											o													o	o				o				o			o	o
Initiation/asking	o			o							o			o	o	o				o									o							o	o
Listening (advanced)	o			o							o			o	o	o				o							o		o							o	o
Answering/responding											o			o	o	o				o									o								o
Topic maintenance														o	o					o									o							o	o
Termination	o													o	o					o									o								
Complimenting																																					
Co-operating	o	o		o							o	o		o	o	o	o	o		o				o	o	o	o		o			o	o		o	o	o
Turn-taking, breaking in	o	o		o							o	o		o	o	o	o	o		o				o	o	o	o		o			o	o		o	o	o
Affective skills																																					
Identification of feelings				o											o	o		o		o	o				o	o		o	o			o		o	o		
Recognizing own feelings				o											o	o		o		o					o	o		o	o			o		o	o		
other's feelings				o											o					o									o			o			o		
Trust																	o	o							o			o							o		
Disclosures	o									o					o									o		o			o								
Cognitive skills																																					
Social perception													o	o	o	o		o		o				o	o	o	o		o			o	o		o	o	o
Problem-solving		o	o											o	o	o		o		o					o	o	o	o			o				o		o
Self-instruction				o	o										o	o									o	o	o										
Self-monitoring, etc.	o			o	o												o	o		o				o		o	o	o			o	o			o		o
Negotiating																	o						o						o								
Assertion	o														o																						

Patient Group: Dysphasia (contd)

EXERCISE NUMBER:	38	39	40	41	42	43	44	45	46	47	48	49	50	51	52	53	54	55	56	57	58	59	60	61	62	63	64	65	66	67	68	69	70	71	72	73	74
Foundation skills																																					
Gelling							o	o									o		o	o					o	o	o				o	o	o		o	o	o
Observation	o		o	o			o	o	o	o							o	o		o			o	o	o	o	o		o	o	o	o	o	o	o	o	o
Eye-contact	o		o	o			o	o	o	o							o	o		o			o		o	o	o		o	o	o	o	o	o	o	o	o
Posture																	o			o			o	o	o		o			o	o	o	o		o		
Presentation/grooming																																					
Facial expression			o	o			o	o	o	o							o		o	o			o	o	o	o				o	o	o	o	o	o	o	o
Gesture			o	o			o	o	o	o							o		o				o	o	o	o	o				o	o	o	o	o	o	o
Space/proximity			o	o			o	o	o	o																					o	o	o	o	o	o	o
Listening (basic)	o		o				o	o	o	o							o	o	o	o			o	o	o	o			o		o	o	o		o	o	
Volume, prosody, etc	o		o				o	o	o	o			o	o			o	o		o			o	o	o	o					o	o	o	o	o		
Relaxation																																					
Touch	o		o				o	o	o								o	o					o	o		o				o	o	o			o	o	
Memory						o	o	o	o								o		o				o		o						o			o	o	o	o
Interaction skills																																					
Greetings	o																						o								o	o	o	o	o	o	o
Initiation/asking	o																	o	o			o			o						o	o	o	o	o	o	
Listening (advanced)	o																					o									o	o	o		o		
Answering/responding	o											o										o	o								o	o	o		o	o	
Topic maintenance																															o	o	o		o		
Termination																																					
Complimenting																															o	o	o		o	o	
Co-operating	o		o			o	o	o									o	o	o			o	o	o	o	o	o			o	o	o	o	o	o	o	o
Turn-taking, breaking in	o					o	o	o		o							o	o	o			o	o	o	o	o	o			o	o	o	o	o	o	o	o
Affective skills																																					
Identification of feelings	o	o																	o				o	o							o	o	o		o	o	
Recognizing own feelings																			o				o	o	o	o					o	o	o		o	o	
other's feelings			o																o						o	o					o	o	o		o	o	
Trust			o																o						o	o					o	o			o		
Disclosures																							o		o												
Cognitive skills																																					
Social perception	o	o															o	o		o			o	o	o	o	o			o	o	o	o		o	o	o
Problem-solving	o	o											o										o	o	o	o					o	o	o	o	o	o	o
Self-instruction									o										o							o					o						
Self-monitoring, etc.																										o					o	o	o		o		
Negotiating										o																						o	o		o		o
Assertion					o																														o		

Patient Group: Dysphasia (contd)

EXERCISE NUMBER:	75	76	77	78	79	80	81	82	83	84	85	86	87	88	89	90	91	92	93	94	95	96	97	98	99	100	101	102	103	104	105	106	107	108	109	110	111	112	113
Foundation skills																																							
Gelling	o			o		o	o	o	o									o		o	o		o	o	o	o	o					o	o				o	o	o
Observation	o		o	o		o	o	o	o				o					o	o	o	o		o	o	o	o	o					o	o		o	o	o	o	
Eye-contact	o					o	o	o	o				o					o	o	o	o		o	o	o	o	o					o	o			o		o	
Posture						o	o		o				o					o	o	o	o		o	o		o	o					o	o						
Presentation/grooming						o																																	
Facial expression	o			o		o	o	o	o				o					o		o	o		o	o	o	o	o					o	o				o	o	
Gesture	o			o		o	o	o	o				o					o		o				o	o	o	o				o	o	o						
Space/proximity	o			o		o	o		o				o							o											o	o							
Listening (basic)	o			o		o	o		o				o					o		o	o		o	o		o	o				o	o	o			o		o	
Volume, prosody, etc	o			o		o	o		o				o					o		o	o		o	o	o	o	o				o	o	o			o		o	
Relaxation																								o															
Touch	o			o		o								o						o	o		o																
Memory	o			o		o					o		o							o	o			o	o	o							o			o	o	o	o
Interaction skills																																							
Greetings	o																				o																		
Initiation/asking	o						o	o			o		o					o	o	o	o		o								o		o						
Listening (advanced)							o						o					o	o												o		o						
Answering/responding											o		o					o				o	o										o						
Topic maintenance											o		o							o	o																		
Termination													o					o	o																				
Complimenting						o	o		o	o	o	o	o					o	o												o	o				o	o		
Co-operating	o			o		o	o		o	o	o	o	o					o	o				o	o							o	o							
Turn-taking, breaking in	o			o		o	o		o	o	o	o	o					o	o	o	o		o									o			o				
Affective skills																																							
Identification of feelings	o						o		o	o	o		o					o	o	o					o	o	o		o		o								
Recognizing own feelings	o						o		o		o		o					o	o						o	o													
other's feelings	o								o		o		o					o							o	o	o		o		o	o							
Trust									o		o		o					o							o	o													
Disclosures	o						o		o		o		o					o						o							o								
Cognitive skills																																							
Social perception	o					o	o		o	o	o	o	o					o											o		o								
Problem-solving						o	o		o	o	o	o	o					o		o				o			o				o		o						o
Self-instruction						o	o		o	o	o	o	o					o				o	o				o				o		o					o	
Self-monitoring, etc.						o	o		o	o	o	o	o					o					o	o							o		o				o	o	
Negotiating						o	o		o	o	o	o	o					o													o		o						
Assertion	o					o	o		o	o	o	o	o					o						o							o		o						o

Patient Group: Learning Disability

EXERCISE NUMBER:	1	2	3	4	5	6	7	8	9	10	11	12	13	14	15	16	17	18	19	20	21	22	23	24	25	26	27	28	29	30	31	32	33	34	35	36	37
Foundation skills																																					
Gelling		o	o	o	o	o	o	o	o	o	o			o	o	o	o			o		o	o	o	o	o	o	o	o	o	o	o	o	o	o	o	o
Observation		o	o	o	o	o	o	o	o	o	o			o	o	o	o			o	o	o	o	o	o	o	o	o	o	o	o	o	o	o	o	o	o
Eye-contact	o			o	o	o	o	o	o	o	o			o	o	o	o	o	o	o	o	o	o	o	o	o	o	o	o	o	o	o	o	o	o	o	o
Posture	o							o			o	o		o	o	o					o			o				o	o	o	o			o			
Presentation/grooming																																					
Facial expression		o	o		o	o	o	o	o	o	o			o	o	o	o	o	o	o	o			o	o	o	o	o	o	o	o	o	o	o	o	o	o
Gesture					o	o	o	o	o	o	o			o	o		o	o	o	o	o			o	o	o			o			o	o			o	o
Space/proximity	o	o	o	o	o				o	o	o			o	o		o	o		o	o			o	o	o	o	o	o	o	o	o	o	o		o	o
Listening (basic)	o	o	o	o	o	o			o	o	o	o		o	o		o	o		o	o	o		o	o	o	o	o	o	o		o	o		o	o	o
Volume, prosody, etc	o	o	o	o		o			o	o	o	o					o			o												o				o	o
Relaxation									o			o	o		o			o		o		o		o	o	o		o	o	o				o				
Touch	o	o				o					o	o									o			o		o		o	o			o	o	o			o
Memory	o	o	o		o			o			o		o	o		o		o		o		o		o	o			o	o								o
Interaction skills																																					
Greetings					o						o			o	o	o	o			o			o	o	o	o			o				o				o
Initiation/asking	o			o							o			o	o	o				o			o				o		o								o
Listening (advanced)	o			o							o				o	o				o									o								o
Answering/responding														o	o		o			o									o								o
Topic maintenance	o						o				o			o			o			o								o									
Termination								o																				o	o								
Complimenting																	o	o	o	o		o			o	o		o	o	o							
Co-operating	o	o			o	o	o				o	o		o	o	o	o	o	o	o			o	o	o	o	o	o	o	o	o	o	o	o	o	o	o
Turn-taking, breaking in	o	o			o						o	o		o	o	o	o	o	o	o			o	o	o	o	o	o	o	o	o	o	o	o	o	o	o
Affective skills																																					
Identification of feelings					o	o	o								o	o	o	o	o	o	o					o	o	o	o	o	o	o	o	o	o		
Recognizing own feelings					o													o	o	o						o	o	o	o	o	o		o			o	o
other's feelings					o		o								o		o	o	o	o						o			o			o					
Trust																	o	o	o							o		o									
Disclosures	o										o				o			o	o									o									
Cognitive skills																																					
Social perception		o	o											o	o	o	o	o	o	o	o				o	o	o	o	o	o	o	o	o	o	o	o	o
Problem-solving		o	o			o									o	o	o			o	o					o	o	o		o	o			o		o	
Self-instruction																o				o						o			o			o					
Self-monitoring, etc.	o				o	o												o		o	o	o		o	o	o	o	o				o					
Negotiating					o																	o															
Assertion	o																																				

Patient Group: Learning Disability (contd)

EXERCISE NUMBER:	38	39	40	41	42	43	44	45	46	47	48	49	50	51	52	53	54	55	56	57	58	59	60	61	62	63	64	65	66	67	68	69	70	71	72	73	74
Foundation skills																																					
Gelling		o	o	o	o	o	o	o	o	o	o	o	o	o		o	o		o				o	o	o	o	o	o	o	o	o	o	o	o	o	o	o
Observation	o	o	o	o	o	o	o	o	o	o	o	o	o	o	o	o	o	o		o			o	o	o	o	o	o	o	o	o	o	o	o	o	o	o
Eye-contact	o	o	o				o	o	o	o	o	o	o	o	o	o	o	o	o	o			o	o	o	o	o	o		o	o	o	o	o	o	o	o
Posture		o	o	o											o																						
Presentation/grooming															o																						
Facial expression	o	o	o				o	o	o	o	o	o		o		o	o	o	o		o	o	o	o	o			o	o	o	o	o	o			o	
Gesture		o	o				o	o	o	o	o										o		o		o		o	o	o		o	o					
Space/proximity												o						o										o									
Listening (basic)	o	o	o				o	o	o	o	o	o		o	o	o	o	o		o			o	o	o	o		o	o	o	o	o					o
Volume, prosody, etc	o	o	o				o	o	o	o	o	o	o	o	o	o	o	o	o	o			o	o	o	o		o		o	o						o
Relaxation	o																																				
Touch					o	o	o	o	o	o	o	o		o	o	o	o	o		o			o	o	o			o	o	o							
Memory	o						o	o											o		o		o											o		o	o
Interaction skills																																					
Greetings	o																		o	o	o	o		o		o					o	o	o	o	o	o	o
Initiation/asking	o																		o	o	o	o		o		o					o	o		o	o		o
Listening (advanced)	o																				o		o	o							o				o		
Answering/responding	o					o																									o						
Topic maintenance																														o	o						o
Termination																																					
Complimenting	o						o	o	o	o	o	o		o		o	o	o	o	o	o		o	o	o	o	o		o	o	o		o				o
Co-operating	o	o				o	o	o	o	o	o	o		o		o	o	o	o	o	o		o	o	o	o	o	o	o	o	o	o	o				o
Turn-taking, breaking in	o	o				o	o	o	o	o	o	o	o	o	o	o	o	o													o	o					
Affective skills																																					
Identification of feelings		o	o																o									o	o	o	o	o		o	o	o	o
Recognizing own feelings																			o					o		o		o		o	o	o		o	o	o	
other's feelings				o															o									o		o	o	o		o	o	o	
Trust																			o			o	o		o	o	o	o	o	o	o	o		o	o	o	
Disclosures																			o					o	o						o	o		o	o		
Cognitive skills																																					
Social perception	o	o	o												o		o	o	o				o	o	o	o		o	o	o	o	o	o	o	o	o	
Problem-solving	o	o	o										o		o	o		o	o				o	o					o		o	o	o	o	o	o	o
Self-instruction									o										o												o						
Self-monitoring, etc.																o			o						o												o
Negotiating															o																						
Assertion	o								o																												

Patient Group: Learning Disability (contd)

EXERCISE NUMBER:	75	76	77	78	79	80	81	82	83	84	85	86	87	88	89	90	91	92	93	94	95	96	97	98	99	100	101	102	103	104	105	106	107	108	109	110	111	112	113
Foundation skills																																							
Gelling	o	o	o	o	o	o	o	o	o	o	o					o	o	o	o	o	o	o	o	o	o	o	o	o	o	o	o	o	o	o	o	o	o	o	o
Observation	o	o	o	o	o	o	o	o	o	o	o	o	o	o	o	o	o	o	o	o	o	o	o	o	o	o	o	o	o	o	o	o	o	o	o	o	o	o	
Eye-contact	o	o	o	o	o	o	o		o	o	o	o	o	o	o	o		o	o		o	o	o	o	o	o	o	o	o	o	o	o	o	o	o				
Posture	o	o		o	o	o	o				o	o	o	o	o	o			o			o				o	o				o	o	o						
Presentation/grooming	o				o																																		
Facial expression	o	o			o	o		o	o		o	o	o	o	o	o	o	o	o		o	o	o	o	o	o	o	o	o	o	o	o	o	o	o	o		o	
Gesture	o	o			o			o	o		o	o	o	o	o			o	o		o	o		o			o	o					o	o					
Space/proximity	o	o	o	o	o	o	o	o	o	o	o	o	o	o	o	o	o	o	o	o	o	o	o	o	o	o	o	o	o	o	o	o	o	o	o	o	o	o	o
Listening (basic)	o	o	o	o	o	o	o	o	o	o	o	o	o	o	o	o	o	o	o	o	o	o	o		o		o			o	o	o	o	o	o	o	o	o	
Volume, prosody, etc	o	o	o	o		o	o	o	o		o	o	o	o		o	o	o	o	o	o	o	o	o	o			o				o	o						o
Relaxation						o																																	
Touch	o	o	o	o	o		o	o	o	o	o	o	o	o	o	o	o	o	o	o	o	o	o	o	o	o	o	o	o	o	o	o	o	o	o				o
Memory		o	o		o	o		o			o	o														o													
Interaction skills																																							
Greetings	o	o			o				o		o	o	o								o		o									o							
Initiation/asking	o	o			o				o	o	o	o		o			o	o	o		o											o	o						
Listening (advanced)											o								o				o	o								o	o						
Answering/responding					o			o	o		o									o		o	o																
Topic maintenance								o	o		o	o											o									o	o						
Termination											o	o																											
Complimenting											o	o	o							o												o	o					o	o
Co-operating	o	o	o	o	o	o	o	o	o	o	o	o	o	o	o	o	o	o	o	o	o	o	o	o	o	o	o	o	o	o	o	o	o	o	o	o			
Turn-taking, breaking in	o	o		o	o	o	o	o	o	o	o	o	o	o	o	o	o	o	o	o	o	o	o										o			o		o	
Affective skills																																							
Identification of feelings	o	o						o	o		o	o	o	o	o	o	o	o	o	o	o	o	o	o	o	o	o	o	o	o	o	o	o						
Recognizing own feelings	o	o						o	o		o	o	o	o	o	o	o	o	o	o	o	o	o	o	o	o	o	o	o	o	o	o	o						
other's feelings	o	o									o	o						o	o		o	o	o	o	o	o	o	o	o	o	o	o	o						
Trust	o			o	o			o			o	o	o	o	o												o	o	o	o	o	o	o	o					
Disclosures	o			o	o			o			o	o	o	o													o	o							o					
Cognitive skills																																							
Social perception	o			o	o			o	o		o	o	o	o	o		o	o	o	o			o	o						o	o	o	o						
Problem-solving	o			o	o			o	o		o	o	o	o		o											o						o						
Self-instruction	o	o	o	o				o	o	o	o	o		o	o	o	o	o	o	o		o	o	o								o	o		o	o	o	o	
Self-monitoring, etc.	o	o		o	o			o	o		o	o	o	o								o	o	o								o	o			o	o	o	
Negotiating						o	o		o		o	o																				o	o						
Assertion	o	o		o	o			o	o		o	o	o	o			o		o	o											o	o							o

Patient Group: Dyspraxia

EXERCISE NUMBER:	1	2	3	4	5	6	7	8	9	10	11	12	13	14	15	16	17	18	19	20	21	22	23	24	25	26	27	28	29	30	31	32	33	34	35	36	37
Foundation skills																																					
Gelling					o					o	o			o	o	o	o					o			o	o	o	o	o	o	o	o	o	o	o	o	o
Observation	o	o	o	o	o	o					o	o	o	o	o	o	o	o	o	o	o		o	o	o	o	o	o	o	o	o	o	o	o	o	o	o
Eye-contact	o	o	o	o	o	o				o	o	o	o	o	o	o	o	o	o	o	o		o	o	o	o	o	o	o	o	o		o	o	o		o
Posture	o			o	o	o				o	o	o	o	o	o	o	o	o	o	o	o	o	o	o	o	o	o	o	o	o	o						
Presentation/grooming												o																	o	o							
Facial expression	o				o	o				o	o	o	o	o	o	o	o	o	o	o	o		o	o	o	o	o	o	o	o		o	o		o		o
Gesture	o				o	o				o	o	o	o	o	o	o		o	o	o	o	o	o	o	o	o		o	o			o	o		o		o
Space/proximity	o	o	o							o	o	o	o	o	o	o	o	o	o	o	o	o	o	o		o	o	o	o	o	o		o	o	o	o	o
Listening (basic)	o	o								o	o	o	o	o	o	o	o	o	o	o	o	o	o	o		o	o					o	o				
Volume, prosody, etc	o									o	o	o	o	o	o	o	o	o	o	o			o	o			o					o	o	o		o	
Relaxation																																					
Touch	o										o	o		o	o	o	o						o	o		o	o	o	o								
Memory	o	o	o							o	o	o	o	o	o	o	o	o	o	o			o	o	o				o	o				o			o
Interaction skills																																					
Greetings											o		o	o	o	o	o							o	o				o								
Initiation/asking		o			o						o		o	o	o	o	o	o	o	o								o	o				o				o
Listening (advanced)											o		o	o	o	o		o	o	o			o				o		o								o
Answering/responding	o			o	o						o			o	o	o		o	o	o			o			o			o	o							o
Topic maintenance														o	o	o	o												o	o							o
Termination														o	o	o		o	o	o									o	o							o
Complimenting																																					
Co-operating	o				o					o	o		o	o	o	o	o	o	o	o	o	o	o	o	o	o	o	o	o	o	o	o	o	o			o
Turn-taking, breaking in	o	o			o					o	o		o	o	o	o	o	o	o	o			o	o	o	o	o	o	o	o	o	o	o	o			o
Affective skills																																					
Identification of feelings				o									o	o	o	o	o	o	o	o	o					o	o	o	o	o		o	o		o		o
Recognizing own feelings				o									o	o	o	o		o	o	o	o					o	o	o	o	o		o			o	o	o
other's feelings				o									o	o	o	o	o	o	o	o								o	o	o					o	o	
Trust	o																o	o										o									
Disclosures	o									o				o			o	o						o		o	o	o	o								
Cognitive skills																																					
Social perception			o		o								o	o	o	o	o	o	o	o	o				o	o	o	o	o	o	o	o	o	o	o	o	o
Problem-solving		o	o								o				o	o	o			o			o			o	o	o		o							
Self-instruction					o									o	o	o	o	o					o			o		o				o					
Self-monitoring, etc.					o									o	o	o	o	o					o						o			o			o		o
Negotiating																					o	o	o	o													
Assertion	o					o								o	o	o	o	o						o									o				

Patient Group: Dyspraxia (contd)

EXERCISE NUMBER:	38	39	40	41	42	43	44	45	46	47	48	49	50	51	52	53	54	55	56	57	58	59	60	61	62	63	64	65	66	67	68	69	70	71	72	73	74
Foundation skills																																					
Gelling			o	o	o				o	o	o	o	o	o	o	o	o	o		o			o		o	o	o	o	o	o	o	o	o	o	o	o	o
Observation	o		o	o	o	o			o	o	o	o	o	o	o	o	o	o		o			o		o	o	o	o	o	o	o	o	o	o	o	o	o
Eye-contact	o		o	o	o				o	o	o	o	o		o		o	o		o			o	o	o	o	o	o	o	o	o	o	o	o	o	o	o
Posture														o	o			o						o					o								
Presentation/grooming	o		o	o	o				o		o				o		o		o	o		o	o	o	o	o			o		o	o			o		o
Facial expression			o	o					o	o	o	o		o		o	o	o				o	o	o	o	o		o		o	o	o	o	o	o	o	
Gesture			o	o	o				o	o	o	o	o	o	o	o	o	o	o			o	o	o	o	o	o	o		o	o	o	o	o	o	o	
Space/proximity	o		o	o					o					o			o			o			o	o			o	o	o		o	o	o		o	o	
Listening (basic)	o		o						o	o	o	o	o	o	o	o	o	o	o	o		o	o	o	o	o		o		o	o	o			o	o	o
Volume, prosody, etc	o								o			o								o			o	o							o	o					
Relaxation																																					
Touch			o	o	o				o		o	o	o	o	o	o			o	o	o	o	o	o	o	o	o	o	o	o	o	o	o	o	o	o	o
Memory	o								o		o	o	o	o	o	o		o	o	o	o	o	o	o	o	o			o	o	o	o	o	o	o		o
Interaction skills																																						
Greetings	o																			o	o				o						o	o		o	o	o	
Initiation/asking	o																		o	o	o					o					o	o	o	o	o	o	
Listening (advanced)	o																		o	o					o						o	o			o		
Answering/responding																														o	o	o					
Topic maintenance																																					
Termination																																					
Complimenting								o	o	o	o	o	o	o	o	o	o	o	o	o	o	o	o	o	o	o		o	o	o	o	o			o	o	o
Co-operating	o		o	o	o	o	o	o	o	o	o	o	o	o	o	o	o	o	o	o	o	o	o	o	o	o		o	o	o	o	o	o	o	o	o	o
Turn-taking, breaking in	o		o	o	o	o	o	o	o	o	o	o	o	o	o	o	o	o	o	o	o	o	o	o	o	o											
Affective skills																																						
Identification of feelings			o	o															o					o	o	o	o	o	o	o	o	o	o	o	o	o	o	o
Recognizing own feelings			o																o					o	o	o	o	o	o	o	o	o	o	o	o	o	o	o
other's feelings																																					
Trust			o		o	o													o							o	o		o	o	o	o					
Disclosures																																					
Cognitive skills																																						
Social perception	o		o	o									o	o				o	o		o			o	o	o	o	o	o	o	o	o	o	o	o	o	o
Problem-solving			o	o			o							o				o						o	o	o		o	o	o	o	o	o	o	o		o
Self-instruction																					o		o		o			o	o		o	o			o		
Self-monitoring, etc.																					o		o		o			o	o		o	o			o	o	
Negotiating																																					
Assertion	o		o	o											o						o				o	o		o			o	o			o		o

Patient Group: Dyspraxia (contd)

EXERCISE NUMBER:	75	76	77	78	79	80	81	82	83	84	85	86	87	88	89	90	91	92	93	94	95	96	97	98	99	100	101	102	103	104	105	106	107	108	109	110	111	112	113
Foundation skills																																							
Gelling	o	o	o	o	o	o	o	o	o	o	o	o	o	o	o	o			o	o	o		o	o	o	o	o	o	o	o		o	o	o	o	o			o
Observation	o	o	o	o	o	o	o	o	o	o	o	o	o	o	o	o			o	o	o		o	o	o	o	o	o	o	o		o	o	o		o		o	
Eye-contact	o	o	o		o	o	o	o	o	o	o	o	o	o	o	o	o	o	o	o			o	o	o	o	o	o	o	o		o	o		o			o	
Posture	o	o			o	o	o	o	o	o	o	o	o	o	o	o	o	o	o	o	o		o		o	o	o	o	o	o		o							
Presentation/grooming	o				o																																		
Facial expression	o	o						o	o	o	o	o	o	o	o	o			o		o		o	o	o	o	o	o	o	o	o	o	o	o				o	
Gesture	o	o				o	o	o	o	o	o	o	o	o	o	o			o	o			o	o		o	o	o	o	o	o	o	o	o			o	o	
Space/proximity	o	o		o	o	o		o	o	o	o	o	o	o	o		o		o	o	o		o		o					o	o	o	o		o	o	o	o	
Listening (basic)	o	o		o	o	o		o	o	o	o	o	o	o	o				o	o			o	o	o	o				o	o	o	o						
Volume, prosody, etc	o							o	o	o	o	o	o	o		o		o	o	o	o		o	o	o				o	o	o	o	o	o	o	o	o	o	o
Relaxation	o																																						
Touch	o	o	o	o	o		o		o	o	o	o	o	o	o	o	o		o	o			o	o	o		o		o	o	o		o	o					
Memory		o																				o			o															o
Interaction skills																																							
Greetings	o	o									o										o	o		o							o	o		o				o	
Initiation/asking	o	o					o	o	o	o	o	o		o	o			o	o	o	o		o								o	o							
Listening (advanced)									o		o			o				o	o	o				o						o	o	o							
Answering/responding				o	o					o												o	o						o										
Topic maintenance				o	o					o																													
Termination										o										o		o																	
Complimenting	o	o	o	o	o			o	o	o	o	o	o	o		o	o	o	o	o			o		o		o	o	o	o	o	o	o						o
Co-operating	o	o	o	o	o			o	o	o	o	o	o	o		o	o	o	o	o			o		o		o	o	o	o	o	o	o	o	o	o	o	o	o
Turn-taking, breaking in	o	o			o	o	o	o	o	o	o	o	o	o	o	o	o	o	o	o	o		o							o	o				o			o	
Affective skills																																							
Identification of feelings	o					o			o	o			o	o		o			o	o				o	o	o			o		o		o	o					
Recognizing own feelings	o					o			o	o			o	o		o			o	o			o	o	o	o			o		o		o	o			o	o	
other's feelings	o					o			o	o			o	o					o	o				o	o	o			o		o								
Trust	o			o		o			o	o	o	o	o	o	o	o			o	o				o	o	o			o				o						
Disclosures	o			o		o			o	o	o	o	o	o		o			o	o						o													
Cognitive skills																																							
Social perception	o					o			o	o	o	o	o	o		o		o	o	o				o	o	o					o			o					
Problem-solving									o	o	o		o														o												
Self-instruction	o	o	o		o	o	o	o	o	o	o	o	o	o		o	o	o	o	o			o	o	o	o			o		o		o	o				o	o
Self-monitoring, etc.	o	o	o		o	o	o	o	o	o	o	o	o	o				o	o	o			o	o							o	o	o		o		o	o	
Negotiating	o				o	o	o	o	o	o	o	o	o																		o	o							
Assertion	o				o	o	o	o	o	o	o	o	o	o		o		o	o	o			o	o							o								o

Patient Group: Dysarthria

EXERCISE NUMBER:	1	2	3	4	5	6	7	8	9	10	11	12	13	14	15	16	17	18	19	20	21	22	23	24	25	26	27	28	29	30	31	32	33	34	35	36	37
Foundation skills																																					
Gelling		o	o		o						o		o	o	o				o	o				o	o	o	o	o	o			o	o	o	o	o	o
Observation		o	o		o						o		o	o	o				o	o				o	o	o	o	o	o			o	o	o	o	o	o
Eye-contact	o	o	o		o						o		o	o	o				o	o				o	o	o	o					o	o	o	o		o
Posture	o				o						o	o	o	o	o					o				o	o	o							o				
Presentation/grooming												o																									
Facial expression	o					o					o	o	o	o	o		o	o	o	o	o			o	o	o	o	o	o			o	o	o			o
Gesture	o				o	o					o	o	o	o	o				o	o	o			o	o	o	o	o	o			o	o	o			o
Space/proximity	o	o	o								o		o	o	o		o	o	o	o	o			o	o	o	o	o	o			o	o	o			o
Listening (basic)	o	o									o								o	o	o			o		o						o	o	o			
Volume, prosody, etc	o										o		o	o	o																						
Relaxation																								o	o												
Touch	o	o									o	o																									
Memory	o	o	o								o	o		o	o				o					o	o	o		o	o						o		o
Interaction skills																																					
Greetings											o													o	o								o				o
Initiation/asking			o		o						o		o		o				o	o							o		o								o
Listening (advanced)					o						o				o				o	o									o								o
Answering/responding														o	o				o	o									o								o
Topic maintenance											o			o	o				o	o									o			o	o				o
Termination	o																																				
Complimenting																	o	o											o			o	o		o		o
Co-operating	o	o			o						o		o	o	o		o	o	o	o				o	o	o	o	o	o			o	o		o		o
Turn-taking, breaking in	o	o			o						o		o	o	o				o	o				o	o	o	o	o	o			o	o				o
Affective skills																																					
Identification of feelings					o										o		o	o	o	o	o			o	o	o	o	o	o			o	o	o		o	o
Recognizing own feelings					o										o		o	o	o	o				o	o	o		o	o			o	o	o	o	o	o
other's feelings					o									o	o					o								o	o								
Trust																			o							o		o	o								
Disclosures	o										o								o																		
Cognitive skills																																					
Social perception														o					o		o			o		o	o	o	o				o		o		o
Problem-solving		o	o									o														o	o					o				o	
Self-instruction					o										o				o							o						o			o		o
Self-monitoring, etc.	o				o														o													o					
Negotiating																								o					o								
Assertion		o																										o									

Patient Group: Dysarthria (contd)

EXERCISE NUMBER:	38	39	40	41	42	43	44	45	46	47	48	49	50	51	52	53	54	55	56	57	58	59	60	61	62	63	64	65	66	67	68	69	70	71	72	73	74
Foundation skills																																					
Gelling																	o	o	o	o				o	o	o	o	o	o		o	o	o	o	o	o	o
Observation	o		o	o				o	o	o							o	o	o	o		o	o	o	o	o	o	o	o	o	o	o	o	o	o	o	o
Eye-contact	o		o	o				o	o	o							o	o	o	o		o	o	o	o	o	o	o	o	o	o	o	o	o	o	o	o
Posture			o	o				o	o	o							o	o	o			o	o	o	o	o	o		o	o	o	o	o	o	o	o	
Presentation/grooming																		o					o														
Facial expression	o		o	o				o	o	o							o	o	o	o		o	o	o	o	o				o	o	o	o	o	o	o	o
Gesture			o	o				o	o	o							o	o	o	o		o	o	o	o	o	o			o	o	o	o	o			
Space/proximity			o	o				o	o								o	o	o			o	o	o		o		o		o	o	o	o	o			
Listening (basic)			o	o				o	o				o				o	o	o	o		o	o	o	o	o	o		o		o	o	o	o	o	o	o
Volume, prosody, etc			o					o	o				o				o	o	o	o		o	o	o	o	o			o		o	o	o	o	o	o	o
Relaxation																																					
Touch																												o				o		o		o	
Memory	o		o					o									o	o	o	o		o	o	o	o	o		o	o	o	o	o	o	o	o	o	o
Interaction skills																																					
Greetings	o																														o	o	o	o	o	o	o
Initiation/asking	o																					o		o							o	o	o	o	o	o	o
Listening (advanced)	o																					o		o	o						o	o	o	o	o	o	
Answering/responding																										o					o	o		o		o		o
Topic maintenance																															o	o						
Termination																															o	o						
Complimenting																													o	o	o	o	o	o	o	o	o
Co-operating	o							o									o	o				o	o	o	o	o	o		o	o	o	o	o	o	o	o	o
Turn-taking, breaking in	o							o									o	o				o	o	o	o	o	o		o		o	o	o	o	o	o	o
Affective skills																																					
Identification of feelings	o	o																	o					o		o		o	o	o	o	o	o	o	o	o	o
Recognizing own feelings	o																		o					o		o		o	o	o	o	o	o	o	o	o	o
other's feelings		o																	o					o		o		o	o	o	o	o	o	o		o	o
Trust																			o						o	o		o	o	o	o	o	o	o	o	o	o
Disclosures																			o			o				o				o	o	o	o	o	o	o	o
Cognitive skills																																					
Social perception	o	o															o	o	o					o	o	o		o		o	o	o	o	o	o	o	o
Problem-solving	o												o				o	o						o	o	o		o			o	o	o				o
Self-instruction				o																			o		o	o				o	o	o	o	o		o	o
Self-monitoring, etc.																			o				o		o						o	o		o		o	
Negotiating																															o	o					
Assertion	o																o	o	o					o		o					o		o		o	o	o

Patient Group: Dysarthria (contd)

EXERCISE NUMBER:	75	76	77	78	79	80	81	82	83	84	85	86	87	88	89	90	91	92	93	94	95	96	97	98	99	100	101	102	103	104	105	106	107	108	109	110	111	112	113
Foundation skills																																							
Gelling	o	o	o	o		o	o	o	o			o	o	o	o			o	o	o	o		o	o	o	o	o	o				o	o	o	o		o	o	o
Observation	o	o	o			o	o	o	o			o	o	o	o			o	o	o	o		o	o	o	o	o	o			o	o	o		o	o	o	o	
Eye-contact	o	o	o			o	o	o	o			o	o	o	o			o	o	o			o	o	o	o	o	o		o	o	o	o	o		o		o	
Posture	o					o			o			o						o	o	o							o	o		o	o	o							
Presentation/grooming	o					o						o	o																										
Facial expression	o	o				o			o	o		o	o	o	o			o	o		o		o	o	o	o	o	o			o	o	o	o					
Gesture	o	o				o			o	o		o	o	o	o		o	o	o				o	o		o	o				o	o		o					
Space/proximity	o	o				o			o	o		o	o	o			o	o	o		o		o	o	o	o	o	o			o	o	o	o	o		o	o	
Listening (basic)	o	o	o	o		o			o	o	o	o	o	o				o	o		o		o	o	o	o	o	o			o	o	o	o	o	o	o	o	
Volume, prosody, etc		o	o						o			o	o	o				o	o		o		o	o			o												
Relaxation																																							
Touch	o	o	o			o	o	o	o			o	o			o		o	o		o		o	o		o	o						o						
Memory		o	o						o			o						o	o		o		o	o									o		o	o			
Interaction skills																																							
Greetings	o	o																				o																	
Initiation/asking	o	o				o	o	o	o			o						o				o	o	o							o	o							
Listening (advanced)									o			o		o				o	o					o							o	o							
Answering/responding																							o																
Topic maintenance								o	o	o		o	o					o	o				o																
Termination								o	o	o		o	o																										
Complimenting	o	o				o	o		o	o		o	o	o				o	o				o	o							o	o			o	o			
Co-operating	o	o				o	o	o	o	o		o	o	o		o		o	o				o	o						o	o	o							
Turn-taking, breaking in	o	o				o	o	o	o	o		o	o	o				o	o		o		o	o									o		o				
Affective skills																																							
Identification of feelings	o	o				o	o		o	o		o	o	o				o	o	o			o		o	o	o				o								
Recognizing own feelings	o	o				o	o		o	o		o	o	o				o	o				o		o	o	o												
other's feelings	o								o	o		o	o	o				o							o	o	o												
Trust	o					o	o		o	o		o	o		o									o					o										
Disclosures	o					o	o		o	o		o	o	o									o	o															
Cognitive skills																																							
Social perception	o					o	o		o	o		o	o	o				o					o	o				o			o								
Problem-solving						o	o		o	o		o	o					o	o				o	o							o					o			
Self-instruction	o					o	o		o	o		o	o	o				o	o				o	o							o	o					o		
Self-monitoring, etc.	o					o	o		o	o		o	o	o				o	o				o	o	o						o	o					o	o	
Negotiating									o			o	o																		o	o							
Assertion	o					o	o		o	o		o	o	o				o	o				o		o														o

Patient Group: Elderly

EXERCISE NUMBER:	1	2	3	4	5	6	7	8	9	10	11	12	13	14	15	16	17	18	19	20	21	22	23	24	25	26	27	28	29	30	31	32	33	34	35	36	37
Foundation skills																																					
Gelling		o	o								o			o					o	o				o	o	o	o	o	o			o	o			o	
Observation		o	o								o	o		o	o				o	o				o	o	o	o	o	o		o	o	o	o		o	o
Eye-contact	o	o	o								o	o	o	o	o	o			o	o	o			o	o	o	o	o	o		o		o	o	o	o	o
Posture	o										o	o	o	o	o				o	o	o			o	o	o	o	o	o								
Presentation/grooming																								o													
Facial expression	o										o	o		o	o		o		o	o	o			o	o	o	o	o	o		o	o	o		o	o	o
Gesture	o										o	o		o			o		o	o	o			o	o	o		o	o				o			o	o
Space/proximity	o	o									o			o	o				o	o	o			o	o				o		o	o	o			o	o
Listening (basic)	o	o									o	o		o	o		o		o	o	o			o			o		o		o	o	o		o	o	o
Volume, prosody, etc	o										o			o	o				o	o	o			o	o				o							o	o
Relaxation													o																								
Touch	o	o									o	o		o										o	o												
Memory	o	o	o								o	o	o	o		o		o		o			o	o	o			o	o								o
Interaction skills																																					
Greetings											o			o	o				o	o				o	o			o					o			o	o
Initiation/asking		o									o				o	o			o	o			o	o			o	o								o	o
Listening (advanced)			o								o				o	o			o	o			o					o								o	o
Answering/responding															o				o	o								o								o	o
Topic maintenance														o	o			o	o									o									
Termination											o				o				o	o								o									
Complimenting																																					
Co-operating		o									o			o	o		o		o	o			o	o	o	o	o	o			o	o	o		o	o	o
Turn-taking, breaking in	o	o									o	o		o	o		o		o	o			o	o	o	o	o	o			o	o	o		o	o	o
Affective skills																																					
Identification of feelings															o		o		o	o	o			o			o	o				o	o	o		o	o
Recognizing own feelings															o		o		o	o						o	o	o			o	o	o	o		o	o
other's feelings															o																	o				o	o
Trust	o										o				o		o		o						o			o									
Disclosures																			o									o									
Cognitive skills																																					
Social perception		o	o											o	o		o		o	o	o			o	o	o	o	o	o			o	o	o		o	o
Problem-solving		o	o									o			o		o																		o		o
Self-instruction	o														o		o		o	o				o	o	o	o				o	o			o	o	o
Self-monitoring, etc.	o														o				o				o						o			o					
Negotiating																								o													
Assertion		o									o			o	o		o		o				o													o	

Patient Group: Elderly (contd)

EXERCISE NUMBER:	38	39	40	41	42	43	44	45	46	47	48	49	50	51	52	53	54	55	56	57	58	59	60	61	62	63	64	65	66	67	68	69	70	71	72	73	74
Foundation skills																																					
Gelling			o				o	o	o		o		o	o			o	o	o	o			o	o	o	o	o			o	o	o	o	o	o	o	o
Observation	o		o				o	o	o	o	o		o	o			o	o	o	o			o	o	o	o	o			o	o	o	o	o	o	o	o
Eye-contact	o		o					o	o	o	o		o	o			o	o	o				o	o	o	o				o	o	o	o	o	o	o	
Posture									o	o	o	o			o		o	o					o							o	o	o	o				
Presentation/grooming																																					
Facial expression	o		o				o	o	o	o	o		o		o		o	o	o				o	o	o	o	o			o	o	o	o	o	o	o	o
Gesture			o				o	o	o	o	o				o			o	o				o	o	o	o				o	o	o	o	o	o	o	
Space/proximity	o		o				o	o	o	o	o		o				o	o	o				o	o	o	o				o	o	o	o	o	o	o	o
Listening (basic)	o		o				o	o	o	o	o		o		o		o	o	o				o	o	o	o				o	o	o	o	o	o	o	o
Volume, prosody, etc	o																																				
Relaxation																																					
Touch																																					
Memory	o		o				o	o	o	o	o		o		o		o			o	o	o	o	o	o	o				o	o	o	o	o	o	o	o
Interaction skills																																					
Greetings	o																				o	o									o	o	o	o	o	o	o	
Initiation/asking	o																			o	o			o							o	o	o	o	o	o		o
Listening (advanced)	o																			o					o						o			o	o	o		
Answering/responding									o																						o							
Topic maintenance																															o	o			o			
Termination																															o	o						
Complimenting																															o	o		o	o	o	o	o
Co-operating	o		o				o	o	o	o	o		o		o		o	o	o	o			o	o	o	o	o			o	o	o	o	o	o	o	o
Turn-taking, breaking in	o		o				o	o	o	o	o				o		o	o	o	o			o	o	o	o	o			o	o	o	o	o	o	o	o
Affective skills																																					
Identification of feelings	o	o																	o					o	o	o				o	o	o	o	o	o	o	
Recognizing own feelings		o																	o					o	o	o				o	o	o	o	o	o	o	
other's feelings																			o												o	o	o	o	o	o	o	
Trust																			o	o			o	o	o				o	o	o	o		o	o		
Disclosures																			o			o								o	o							
Cognitive skills																																					
Social perception	o	o											o	o			o	o		o				o	o	o				o	o	o	o	o	o	o	
Problem-solving	o	o											o	o			o	o						o	o	o				o	o	o	o	o	o	o	
Self-instruction								o															o	o	o					o	o	o	o	o	o	o	o
Self-monitoring, etc.																															o	o						
Negotiating																																					
Assertion	o							o									o		o	o						o					o	o	o	o	o		o

Patient Group: Elderly (contd)

EXERCISE NUMBER:	75	76	77	78	79	80	81	82	83	84	85	86	87	88	89	90	91	92	93	94	95	96	97	98	99	100	101	102	103	104	105	106	107	108	109	110	111	112	113
Foundation skills																																							
Gelling	o		o			o	o	o	o	o								o	o	o	o	o	o	o	o	o	o	o	o	o	o	o	o			o	o	o	o
Observation	o	o				o	o	o	o	o								o	o	o	o	o	o	o	o	o	o	o	o	o	o	o	o			o	o	o	
Eye-contact	o					o	o	o	o									o	o	o	o	o	o	o	o	o	o	o	o	o	o	o	o			o			
Posture						o	o		o	o	o	o	o	o				o	o	o	o	o	o	o	o	o	o	o	o	o	o		o						
Presentation/grooming						o	o						o																										
Facial expression	o					o	o	o	o	o	o	o	o					o	o	o	o	o	o		o	o	o	o	o	o	o	o	o			o			
Gesture	o					o	o	o	o	o	o	o	o						o	o	o	o		o	o	o	o	o		o	o								
Space/proximity	o					o	o		o	o	o	o	o											o						o	o								
Listening (basic)	o	o				o	o	o	o	o	o	o	o			o		o	o	o	o	o	o	o	o	o	o	o	o	o	o	o	o			o	o	o	o
Volume, prosody, etc	o	o				o	o		o	o	o	o	o			o		o	o	o	o	o	o	o	o	o	o	o	o	o	o	o	o			o	o	o	o
Relaxation																				o				o	o														
Touch	o	o										o																											
Memory	o	o				o				o	o	o				o		o	o	o	o	o	o	o	o	o	o	o				o	o			o	o	o	o
Interaction skills																																							
Greetings	o															o				o	o																		
Initiation/asking	o					o	o		o							o		o	o	o	o	o		o						o		o	o			o			
Listening (advanced)							o		o							o		o	o	o	o	o	o	o						o		o	o			o	o		
Answering/responding									o													o	o																
Topic maintenance						o			o	o													o	o															
Termination						o			o	o												o	o																
Complimenting						o	o		o	o	o	o																											
Co-operating	o	o				o	o		o	o	o	o	o	o				o	o	o								o	o		o	o				o	o	o	
Turn-taking, breaking in	o	o				o	o		o	o	o	o	o	o				o	o	o	o		o		o								o				o		
Affective skills																																							
Identification of feelings	o	o				o			o	o	o	o						o	o	o	o			o		o	o	o	o	o	o		o						
Recognizing own feelings	o	o				o	o			o	o	o						o	o	o	o			o		o	o	o	o	o	o		o						
other's feelings	o										o	o	o						o	o				o		o	o	o	o	o	o		o						
Trust	o					o			o	o	o	o						o	o	o	o			o		o	o	o	o	o									
Disclosures	o					o			o	o	o	o						o	o	o	o		o	o		o	o	o	o	o									
Cognitive skills																																							
Social perception						o	o		o	o	o	o						o	o	o		o	o	o															
Problem-solving						o	o		o	o	o	o						o	o	o		o	o	o		o				o		o				o	o		
Self-instruction						o	o		o	o	o	o				o		o	o	o	o	o	o								o					o			
Self-monitoring, etc.						o	o		o	o	o	o						o	o	o		o	o	o						o		o							
Negotiating						o			o	o	o	o						o	o					o	o								o						
Assertion	o					o	o		o	o	o	o						o	o	o										o	o		o						o

Patient Group: Language Impairment

EXERCISE NUMBER:	1	2	3	4	5	6	7	8	9	10	11	12	13	14	15	16	17	18	19	20	21	22	23	24	25	26	27	28	29	30	31	32	33	34	35	36	37
Foundation skills																																					
Gelling	o	o	o		o	o	o	o	o	o	o			o	o		o		o	o	o	o	o	o	o	o	o	o	o	o	o	o	o	o	o	o	o
Observation	o	o	o		o	o	o	o	o	o	o			o	o	o	o		o	o	o	o	o	o	o	o	o	o	o	o	o	o	o	o	o	o	o
Eye-contact	o	o	o	o	o	o	o	o	o	o	o			o	o	o	o		o	o	o	o	o	o	o	o	o	o	o	o	o						
Posture	o				o			o	o	o	o			o	o		o			o		o	o	o		o				o							
Presentation/grooming											o						o			o				o				o	o	o							o
Facial expression	o				o	o			o		o			o	o	o	o	o	o	o	o		o	o	o	o	o	o	o	o	o	o	o	o	o	o	o
Gesture	o				o	o		o	o		o			o	o		o	o		o	o		o	o	o	o				o	o		o	o	o		o
Space/proximity	o	o	o	o		o			o		o			o	o	o	o			o	o		o			o	o			o	o	o					o
Listening (basic)	o	o	o	o			o		o		o			o	o		o			o	o		o	o	o	o	o			o	o		o				o
Volume, prosody, etc	o					o			o		o			o			o			o	o						o										
Relaxation						o		o	o			o																o									
Touch	o							o				o					o						o	o	o			o	o								
Memory	o	o	o								o	o	o	o	o	o	o	o		o			o	o		o		o	o	o	o						o
Interaction skills																																					
Greetings											o		o	o	o	o	o							o	o		o	o	o	o			o				o
Initiation/asking	o		o		o						o				o	o	o		o	o		o	o				o	o	o								o
Listening (advanced)	o			o							o				o	o			o	o		o						o	o								o
Answering/responding											o			o	o	o	o		o	o								o	o								o
Topic maintenance	o													o	o	o	o			o								o	o	o							
Termination	o							o			o			o	o			o										o	o								
Complimenting															o	o	o		o	o			o					o	o			o	o	o	o	o	o
Co-operating	o	o	o		o						o			o	o	o	o	o	o	o		o	o	o	o	o	o	o	o	o	o	o	o	o	o	o	o
Turn-taking, breaking in	o	o	o		o						o	o		o	o	o	o	o	o	o	o	o	o	o	o	o	o	o	o	o	o	o	o	o	o	o	o
Affective skills																																					
Identification of feelings				o							o			o	o		o	o	o	o	o			o	o	o	o	o	o	o		o	o		o		
Recognizing own feelings				o			o								o	o	o	o	o	o						o		o	o	o		o	o	o	o	o	
other's feelings				o											o	o		o	o	o						o		o	o	o							
Trust																	o	o							o			o	o								
Disclosures	o										o										o							o	o								
Cognitive skills																																					
Social perception		o	o			o						o		o	o	o	o	o	o	o	o			o		o	o	o	o	o		o	o		o		o
Problem-solving																										o	o			o							
Self-instruction				o	o													o		o		o							o			o				o	
Self-monitoring, etc.	o			o	o																			o				o	o			o					
Negotiating															o														o								
Assertion	o	o					o																										o		o		o

Patient Group: Language Impairment (contd)

EXERCISE NUMBER:	38	39	40	41	42	43	44	45	46	47	48	49	50	51	52	53	54	55	56	57	58	59	60	61	62	63	64	65	66	67	68	69	70	71	72	73	74
Foundation skills																																					
Gelling			o	o	o	o	o	o	o	o	o	o		o	o	o	o	o	o	o			o	o	o	o	o	o	o	o	o	o	o	o	o	o	o
Observation	o	o	o	o	o	o	o	o	o	o	o	o	o	o	o	o	o	o	o	o	o	o	o	o	o	o	o	o	o	o	o	o	o	o	o	o	o
Eye-contact	o	o	o	o					o	o	o	o	o	o	o	o	o	o	o	o	o	o	o	o	o	o	o	o	o	o	o	o	o	o	o	o	o
Posture														o	o		o	o																			
Presentation/grooming	o											o			o		o		o													o					
Facial expression	o	o	o		o				o	o	o	o		o		o	o	o	o	o	o	o	o	o	o	o		o		o	o	o	o	o	o	o	o
Gesture	o	o	o	o					o	o	o	o				o		o	o	o	o	o	o	o	o	o			o		o	o	o	o	o	o	o
Space/proximity	o	o		o					o	o	o	o	o	o	o												o	o	o							o	o
Listening (basic)	o	o							o	o	o	o		o	o	o	o	o	o	o	o	o	o	o	o	o		o		o	o	o	o	o	o	o	o
Volume, prosody, etc	o	o							o	o		o	o		o	o	o	o	o	o	o	o	o	o	o	o		o		o	o	o	o	o	o	o	o
Relaxation			o																																		
Touch	o	o	o	o	o	o	o	o	o	o	o	o	o	o	o	o	o	o	o	o	o	o	o	o	o	o	o	o	o		o	o	o		o	o	o
Memory	o				o	o	o	o	o	o	o	o	o	o	o	o	o			o	o							o	o	o	o	o	o		o		o
Interaction skills																																					
Greetings	o																		o		o			o	o			o	o	o	o	o	o	o	o	o	o
Initiation/asking	o																		o		o		o		o			o	o	o	o	o	o	o	o	o	o
Listening (advanced)	o																		o			o		o				o	o	o	o	o	o	o	o	o	
Answering/responding	o							o																					o		o	o					
Topic maintenance																														o	o	o				o	
Termination																															o	o					
Complimenting																																				o	
Co-operating	o			o	o	o	o	o	o	o	o	o	o	o	o	o	o	o	o	o	o	o	o	o	o	o	o	o	o	o	o	o	o	o	o	o	o
Turn-taking, breaking in	o				o		o	o	o	o	o	o		o	o	o	o	o	o	o	o	o	o	o	o	o	o	o	o	o	o	o	o	o	o	o	o
Affective skills																																					
Identification of feelings		o	o													o	o		o						o			o	o	o	o	o			o	o	o
Recognizing own feelings																	o		o			o		o				o	o	o	o	o			o	o	o
other's feelings			o																									o	o		o	o			o	o	o
Trust					o														o		o		o		o				o	o	o				o	o	
Disclosures																o	o		o					o		o			o	o	o	o					
Cognitive skills																																					
Social perception	o	o	o	o													o	o	o	o					o	o		o	o	o	o	o	o	o	o	o	o
Problem-solving		o	o						o				o		o		o				o			o	o	o					o	o			o	o	o
Self-instruction																				o			o		o					o	o				o	o	o
Self-monitoring, etc.										o									o												o	o					
Negotiating							o									o																					
Assertion	o								o																o							o			o	o	o

Patient Group: Language Impairment (contd)

EXERCISE NUMBER:	75	76	77	78	79	80	81	82	83	84	85	86	87	88	89	90	91	92	93	94	95	96	97	98	99	100	101	102	103	104	105	106	107	108	109	110	111	112	113
Foundation skills																																							
Gelling	o	o	o	o	o	o	o	o	o	o		o	o	o	o	o	o	o	o	o			o	o	o	o	o	o	o	o	o	o	o	o	o	o	o	o	o
Observation	o	o	o	o	o	o	o	o	o	o		o	o	o	o	o	o	o	o	o	o	o	o	o	o	o	o	o	o	o	o	o	o	o	o	o	o	o	
Eye-contact	o	o	o	o	o	o	o	o	o	o		o	o	o	o	o	o	o	o	o		o	o	o	o	o	o	o	o	o	o	o	o	o	o				
Posture	o			o	o	o	o	o	o	o		o	o	o	o	o	o	o	o	o						o	o												
Presentation/grooming	o					o							o	o					o																				
Facial expression	o	o				o	o	o	o	o		o	o	o	o	o	o	o	o	o			o	o		o	o	o	o	o	o	o	o	o					
Gesture	o	o					o	o	o	o		o	o	o	o		o	o	o				o	o		o	o	o	o	o	o	o	o	o					
Space/proximity	o	o		o	o	o	o	o	o	o	o	o	o	o	o	o	o		o	o	o		o	o		o	o	o	o	o	o	o	o		o	o			
Listening (basic)	o	o		o	o	o	o	o	o	o	o	o	o	o	o	o	o		o	o			o			o	o	o	o	o	o	o	o		o	o			
Volume, prosody, etc	o	o	o			o	o		o	o	o	o	o	o		o		o	o	o	o	o	o	o	o	o	o	o			o	o	o		o	o		o	o
Relaxation										o																													
Touch	o		o	o		o				o		o	o	o	o	o	o	o	o	o	o		o	o	o	o	o	o	o		o	o	o	o		o	o	o	o
Memory	o	o				o				o		o	o							o									o											
Interaction skills																																							
Greetings	o									o		o									o	o																		
Initiation/asking	o	o					o	o	o	o		o	o	o			o	o					o							o	o								
Listening (advanced)												o	o	o			o	o					o								o	o					o			
Answering/responding								o	o	o		o	o	o					o			o																	
Topic maintenance								o	o	o		o	o	o					o			o																	
Termination												o	o						o		o																		
Complimenting												o	o						o											o	o			o	o				
Co-operating	o	o					o	o	o	o		o	o	o	o		o	o	o	o			o							o	o			o					
Turn-taking, breaking in	o	o				o	o	o	o	o		o	o	o			o	o	o	o			o											o					
Affective skills																																							
Identification of feelings	o						o	o		o		o	o	o					o	o						o	o	o		o			o						
Recognizing own feelings	o						o	o		o		o	o	o					o	o						o	o	o		o			o						
other's feelings	o									o		o	o	o					o	o						o	o	o					o						
Trust	o								o	o		o	o						o	o			o			o	o	o											
Disclosures	o								o	o		o	o	o	o				o	o				o		o	o	o					o						
Cognitive skills																																							
Social perception	o						o	o		o		o	o	o		o			o			o	o							o	o			o					
Problem-solving	o						o	o		o		o	o													o													
Self-instruction			o			o	o	o	o	o		o	o	o		o		o	o			o	o							o	o			o			o	o	
Self-monitoring, etc.	o						o	o		o		o	o	o					o			o	o	o						o	o			o					
Negotiating										o		o	o						o										o			o								
Assertion	o					o		o	o	o		o	o	o	o	o	o	o	o					o						o			o						o

References

ADAMS, C AND BISHOP, DVM (1989) Conversational characteristics of children with semantic–pragmatic disorder 1: Exchange structure, turn-taking, repairs and cohesion. British Journal of Disorders of Communication 24, 211 – 39.

APPLE, M (1982) Cultural and Economic Reproduction in Education. London: Routledge and Kegan Paul.

ARGYLE M (1969) Social Interaction. New York: Aldine-Atherton.

ARGYLE, M (1975) Bodily Communication. London: Methuen.

ARGYLE M (1982) The contribution of social interaction research to social skills training, in Wine, JW and Syme MD (Eds.) Social Competence. New York: Guilford Press.

ARGYLE M, FURNHAM A AND GRAHAM J (1981) Social Situations. Cambridge: Cambridge University Press.

ARGYLE M and KENDON A (1967) The experimental analysis of social behaviour, in Berkowitz L (Ed.) Advances in Experimental Social Psychology, 3, 59 – 68.

ASHER, SR, ODEN SL and GOTTMAN JM (1977) Children's friendships in school settings, in Katz LG (Ed.) Current Topics in Early Childhood Education (Vol. 1). Norwood: Ablex.

AUTHIER J, GUSTAFSON K, FIX A and DAUGHTON D (1981) Social skills training: An initial approach, Professional Psychology, 12, 438 – 45.

BALES RF (1950) Interaction Process Analysis: A method for the study of small groups. Cambridge, Mass: Addison-Wesley.

BANDURA A (1969) Principles of Behavior Modification. New York: Holt, Rinehart and Winston.

BANDURA A (1973) Aggression: A Social Learning Analysis. Englewood Cliffs: Prentice-Hall.

BANDURA A (1977) Social Learning Theory. Englewood Cliffs: Prentice-Hall.

BEAZLEY S (1992) Social skills group work with deaf people, in Fawcus M (Ed.) Group Encounters in Speech and Language Therapy. Far Communication Disorders. 63 – 75.

BECK AT (1963) Thinking and depression: I. Idiosyncratic content and cognitive distortions. Archives of General Psychiatry, 9, 36 – 46.

BECK AT (1964) Thinking and depression: II. Theory and therapy. Archives of General Psychiatry, 10, 561 – 71.

BECK AT (1970) Cognitive therapy: Nature and relation to behavior therapy. Behavior Therapy, 1, 184–200.

BECK AT (1976) Cognitive therapy and the emotional disorders. New York: International University Press.

BECK AT, RUSH AJ, SHAW BF and EMERY G (1979) Cognitive therapy of depression. New York: Guilford Press.

BELLACK AS (1987) Social skills training for the treatment of chronic schizophrenics, in Strauss JS, Boker W and Brenner HD (Eds.) Psychological Treatment of Schizophrenia. Bern: Huber, 118 – 25.

BELLACK AS and HERSEN M (Eds.) (1979) Research and Practice in Social Skills Training. New York: Plenum.

BERGER PL and LUCKMANN T (1966) The Social Construction of Reality. Harmondsworth: Penguin.

BIRDWHISTELL R (1970) Kinetics and Context. Philadelphia: University of Pennsylvania Press.

BISHOP DVM and ADAMS C (1989) Conversational characteristics of children with semantic–pragmatic disorder II: What features lead to a judgement of inappropriacy? British Journal of Disorders of Communication 24, 241 – 63.

BLOODSTEIN O (1995) A Handbook on Stuttering. California: Singular Press.

BROOKS-GUNN J and LEWIS M (1985) Temperament and Affective Interaction in Handicapped Infants. Topics in Early Childhood.

BROWN A (1986) Groupwork. Aldershot: Gower.

BRUCH M (1981) A task analysis of assertive behaviour revisited: Replication and extension. Behaviour Therapy, 12, 217 – 30.

BRUCH M, HEISLER B and CONROY C (1981) Effects of conceptual complexity on assertive behaviour. Journal of Counseling Psychology, 28, 377 – 85.

CARTLEDGE G and MILBURN JF (Eds.) (1986) Teaching Social Skills to Children. Innovative Approaches, 2nd Ed. New York: Pergamon Press.

CHANG B (1978) Perceived situational control of daily activities: A new tool. Research in Nursing and Health, 1, 181 – 8.

CHANG M (1970) A study of student teacher reactions to microteaching. Dissertation Abstracts International, 2226A.

CHRISTOFF KA, SCOTT WON, KELLEY ML, SCHLUNDT D, BAER G and KELLEY JA (1985) Social skills and social problem-solving training for shy young adolescents. Behavior Therapy, 16, 468 – 77.

COOKE TP and APOLLONI T (1976) Developing positive social–emotional behaviors: A study of training and generalization effects. Journal of Applied Behavior Analysis, 65 – 78.

CORSINI RJ (1966) Roleplaying in Psychotherapy: A Manual. Chicago: Aldine.

COWEN, EL, PEDERSON A, BABIGIAN H, IZZO LD and TROST MA (1973) Long term follow-up of early detected vulnerable children. Journal of Consulting and Clinical Psychology, 41, 438 – 46.

CROSSMAN ER (1960) Automation and Skill. DSIR Problems of Progress in Industry, No. 9. London: HMSO.

CURRAN JP (1979) Social skills: Methodological issues and future directions, in Bellack AS and Hersen M (Eds.) Research and Practice in Social Skills Training. New York: Plenum.

CURRAN JP and MONTI MP (Eds.) (1982) Social Skills Training. A Practical Handbook for Assessment and Treatment. New York: The Guilford Press.

CURRY M and BROMFIELD C (1994) Personal and Social Education for Primary Schools through Circle Time. NASEN.

DANIELSON J and SAMPSON L (1992) Question the Information: Techniques for Classroom Listening. East Moline: Linguisystems.

DAVIS JM (1986) Effects of mild to moderate hearing impairments in language, educational and psychosocial behaviour in children. Journal of Speech and Hearing Disorders, 51, 53 – 62.

DICKSON DA, HARGIE O, MORROW N (1993) Communication Skills Training for Health Professionals: An Instructors Hand Book. London: Chapman & Hall.

DODGE KA (1985) Facets of social interaction and the assessment of social competence in children. In Schneider B, Rubin K and Ledingham J (Eds.) Children's peer relations: Issues in Assessment and Intervention. New York: Springer-Verlag, 3 – 22.

DOYLE AB (1982) Friends, acquaintances, and strangers: The influence of family. Ethnolinguistic background on social interaction in peer relationship and social skills in childhood, in Rubin KH and Ross HS (Eds.) Peer Relationships and Social Skills in Childhood. New York: Springer.

D'ZURILLA TJ (1986) Problem-solving therapy: A social competence approach to clinical intervention. New York: Springer.

D'ZURILLA TJ (1988) Problem-solving therapies. In Dobson KS (Ed.) Handbook of Cognitive–behavioral Therapies. New York: Guilford, 85 – 135.

EISLER RM, MILLER PM and HERSEN M (1973) Components of assertive behavior. Journal of Clinical Psychology, 29, 295 – 9.

ELLIS A (1962) Reason and Emotion in Psychotherapy. Secaucus. NJ: Citadel.

ELLIS A (1975) How to Live with a Neurotic. Rev. ed. North Hollywood, CA: Wilshire Books.

ELLIS A (1996) Better, Deeper, and More Enduring Brief Therapy: The Rational Emotive Behavior Therapy Approach. New York:Brunner/Mazel.

ELLIS R and WHITTINGTON D (1981) A Guide to Social Skills Training. Beckenham: Croom Helm.

EYSENCK HJ (1952) The effects of psychotherapy: An evaluation. Journal of Consulting Psychology, 16, 319.

FAIRBANKS G and PROVONOST W (1939) An experimental study of the pitch charac- teristics of the voice during the expression of emotion. Speech Monographs, 6, 87 – 104.

FALLOON IRH, HAHLWEG K and TARRIER N (1990) Family interventions in the community management of schizophrenia: Methods and results, in Straube ER and Hahlweg K (Eds.) Schizophrenia, Concepts, Vulnerability and Inter- ventions. Berlin: Springer, 217 – 40.

FISHER R (1990) Teaching Children to Think. Cheltenham: Stanley Thornes.

FROSH S (1983) Children and teachers in school, in Spence S and Shepherd G Developments in Social Skills Training. New York: Academic Press.

FURNHAM A (1983) Editorial introduction. Research in social skills training: A critique, in Ellis R and Whittington D (Eds.) New Directions in Social Skills Training. London: Croom Helm.

FURNHAM A (1985) Social skills training. A European perspective, in L'Abate L and Milan MA (Eds.) Handbook of Social Skills Training and Research. New York: Wiley.

FURNHAM A (1986) Social skills training with adolescents and young adults, in Hollin CR and Trower P (Eds.) Handbook of Social Skills Training. Inter- national Series in Experimental Psychology, Vol. 12. Oxford: Pergamon Press.

FURNHAM A and PENDRED J (1983) Attitudes towards the mentally and physically disabled. British Journal of Medical Psychology, 56, 170 – 87.

GAMBRILL E (1984) Social skills training, in Dale (ed.) Teaching Psychological Skills. Belmont, CA: Brooks/Cole Publishing Company. 104 – 30.

GARFIELD SL and BERGIN AE (Eds.) (1986) Handbook of Psychotherapy and Behavior Change. New York: Wiley.

GLENWICK DS and JASON LA (1984) Locus of intervention in child cognitive behavior therapy, in Meyers AW and Craighead WE (Eds.) Cognitive Behavior Therapy with Children. New York: Plenum Press.

GOLDSTEIN AP, SPRAFKIN RP, GERSHAW NJ and KLEIN P (1980) Skill-streaming the Adolescent. A Structured Learning Approach to Teaching Prosocial Skills. Illinois: Research Press Company.

GOLDSTEIN H and GALLAGHER TM (1992) Strategies for promoting the social–communicative competence of young children with specific language impairment, in Odom SL, McConnell, SR and McEvoy MA (Eds.) Social Competence of Young Children with Disabilities: Issues and Strategies for Intervention. Baltimore: Brookes, 93 – 109.

GOLDSTEIN H and RAEKE FERRELL D (1987) Augmenting communicative interaction between handicapped and nonhandicapped preschool children. Journal of Speech and Hearing Disorders, 52, 200 – 11.

GOTTLIEB J and DAVIS JE (1973) Social acceptance of EMRs during overt behavioral interaction. American Journal of Mental Deficiency, 78, 141 – 3.

GRAHAM J and HEYWOOD S (1976) The effects of elimination of hand gestures and of verbal codability on speech performance. European Journal of Social Psychology, 5, 189 – 95.

GRAWE K (1997) 'Moderne' Verhaltenstherapie oder allgemeine psychotherapie? Verhaltenstherapie und Verhaltensmedizin, 18. (2). 137 – 59.

GREENBERGER D and PADESKY C (1995) Mind over mood: A cognitive therapy treatment manual for clients. New York: Guilford Press.

GRESHAM FM (1981) Social skills training with handicapped children: A review. Review of Educational Research, 51, 139 – 76.

GRICE PP (1967) Logic and conversation, in Cole P and Morgan JL (Eds.) Syntax and Semantics III: Speech Acts. New York: Academic Press.

GROCE N (1985) Everyone Here Spoke Sign Language: Hereditary Deafness on Martha's Vineyard. London: Harvard University Press.

GURALNICK MJ (1992) A hierarchical model for understanding children's peer-related social competence. In Odom SL, McConnell SR and McEvoy MA (Eds.) Social Competence of Young Children with Disabilities: Issues and Strategies for Intervention. Baltimore: Brookes, 37 – 64.

HALL ET (1959) The Silent Language. New York: Doubleday.

HALL ET (1966) The Hidden Dimension. New York: Doubleday.

HARGIE D, SAUNDERS C and DICKSON D (1981) Social Skills in Interpersonal Communication, Beckenham: Croom Helm.

HARGIE O, SAUNDERS C AND DICKSON D (1994) Social Skills in Interpersonal Communication. London: Routledge.

HARPER RG, WIENS AN and MATARAZZO JD (1978) Nonverbal Communication: The State of the Art. New York: Wiley.

HAYES C (1997) Applying Personal Construct Psychology. In France J and Muir N (Eds.) Communication and the Mentally Ill Patient: Developmental and Linguistic Approaches to Schizophrenia. London: Jessica Kingsley.

HEATHERINGTON M (1989) Listening and talking in year one. In Dwyer J (ed.), A Sea of Talk. Rozelle: Primary English Teaching Association, 9–20.

HITCHINGS A and SPENCE R (1991) The Personal Communication Plan for people with Learning Disabilities. Windsor: NFER – Nelson.

HOGARTY GE, ANDERSON CM, REISS DJ, KORNBLITH SJ, GREENWALD DP, JAVNA CD,

MADONIA MJ (The EPICS Schizophrenia Research Group) (1986) Family psychoeducation, social skills training and maintenance chemotherapy in the aftercare treatment of schizophrenia: I. One year effects of a controlled study on relapse and expressed emotion. Archives of General Psychiatry 43, 633 – 42.

HOGARTY GE and ANDERSON C (1987) A controlled study of family therapy, social skills training and maintenance chemotherapy in the aftercare treatment of schizophrenic patients: Preliminary effects on relapse and expressed emotion at one year, in Strauss JS, Boker W and Brenner HD (Eds.) Psychosocial Treatment of Schizophrenia. Bern: Huber.

HOLLIN CR and TROWER P (1986) Social skills training: a retrospective analysis and summary of applications, in Hollin CR and Trower R (Eds.) Handbook of Social Skills Training. Applications across the Life-span, (Vol. 1). Oxford: Pergamon Press.

HONEY P (1988) Face to Face: A Practical Guide to Interactive Skill. Aldershot: Gaver.

HOPPER R and WILLIAMS F (1973) Speech characteristics and employability. Speech Monographs, 40, 296 – 302.

HOPS H (1983) Children's social competence and skill: Current research practices and future directions. Behavior Therapy, 14, 3 – 18.

JACOBSON E (1938) Progressive Relaxation. Chicago: University of Chicago Press.

JACOBSON L (1981) The role of inanimate objects in early peer interaction. Child Development, 52, 618 – 26.

JOHNSON GO (1950) A study of social position of mentally handicapped children in the regular grades. American Journal of Mental Deficiency, 55, 60 – 89.

JUSTER HR, HEIMBERG RG and HOLT CS (1997) Social phobia: Diagnostic issues and review of cognitive behavioral treatment, in Hersen M, Eisler RN and Miller PM (Eds.) Progress in Behavior Modification. Pacific Grove/CA: Brooks/Cole.

KAGAN J (1984) The Nature of the Child. New York: Basic Books.

KAZDIN A and HERSEN M (1980) The current status of behaviour therapy. Behaviour Modification, 4, 283 – 302.

KELLY A (1996) Talk about a Social Communication Skills Package. Bicester, Oxon: Winslow Press.

KELLY J, KERN J, KIRKLEY B et al. (1980) Reactions to assertive versus unassertive behavior: Differential effects for males and females and implications for assertiveness training. Behavior Therapy, 11, 670 – 82.

KENDALL PC and BRASWELL L (1985) Cognitive–behavioral Therapy for Impulsive Children. New York: The Guilford Press.

KLECK R (1969) Physical stigma and task orientated interaction. Human Relations, 22, 51 – 60.

KNAUS WJ (1974) Rational Emotive Education. New York: Institute for Rational Living.

L'ABATE L and MILAN MA (Eds.) (1985) Handbook of Social Skills Training and Research. New York: Wiley.

LADD GW and MIZE J (1983) A cognitive-social learning model of social skills training. Psychological Review, 10, 127 – 57.

LANG PJ (1993) The three-system approach to emotion, in Birbaumer N and Öhman A (Eds.) The Structure of Emotion. Seattle: Hogrefe and Huber. 18–30.

LEFKOWITZ MR, BLAKE R and MOUTON J (1955) Status factors in pedestrian violation of traffic signals. Journal of Abnormal and Social Psychology, 51, 704 – 6.

LEMANEK KL, WILLIAMSON DA, GRESHAM FM and JENSEN BJ (1986) Social skills training with hearing-impaired children and adolescents. Behaviour Modification, 10, 55 – 71.

LEWIN K, LIPPITT R and WHITE RK (1939) Patterns of aggressive behavior in experimentally created social climates. Journal of Social Psychology, 10, 271 – 99.

LIBERMAN RP, VAUGHN C, AITCHISON RA and FALLOON I (1977) Social Skills Training for Relapsing Schizophrenics. National Institute of Mental Health.

LIBET JM and LEWINSOHN PM (1973) Concept of social skill with special reference to the behavior of depressed persons. Journal of Consulting and Clinical Psychology, 40, 304 – 12.

LUCOCK MP and SALKOVSKIS PM (1988) Cognitive factors in social anxiety and its treatment. Behaviour Research and Therapy, 26, 297 – 302.

LURIA AR (1961) The Role of Speech in the Regulation of Normal and Abnormal Behaviors. New York: Liverwright.

MANCUSO R (1988) Question the Direction: A Program for Teaching Careful Listening and the Questioning of Unclear Directions. East Moline: Linguisystems.

MANN RA (1976) Assessment of behavioral excesses in children, in Hersen M and Bellack AA (Eds.) Behavioral Assessment: A Practical Handbook. Elmsford: Pergamon Press.

MARKOVITS H and STRAYER FF (1982) Toward an applied social ethology: A case study of social skills among blind children, in Rubin KH and Ross HS (Eds.) Peer Relationships and Social Skills in Childhood. New York: Springer.

MARZILLIER JS and WINTER K (1978) Success and failure in social skills training: Individual differences. Behaviour Research and Therapy, 16, 67 – 84.

MATSON J, KAZDIN A and ESVELDT-DAWSON K (1980) Training interpersonal skills among mentally retarded and socially dysfunctional children. Behaviour Research and Therapy, 18, 419 – 27.

MATSON JL and DI LORENZO TM (1986) Social skills training and mental handicap and organic impairment, in Hollin CR and Trower P (Eds.) Handbook of Social Skills Training. Clinical Applications and New Directions. (Vol. 2). New York: Pergamon Press, 67 – 90.

MATTHEWS WS and BROOKS-GUNN J (1984) Social development in childhood, in Meyers AW and Craighead WE (Eds.) Cognitive Behavior Therapy with Children. New York: Plenum Press.

MAULTSBY MC JR, and ELLIS A (1974) Technique for using Rational–Emotive Imagery. New York: Institute for Rational–Emotive Therapy.

MCFALL R (1982) A review and reformulation of the concept of social skills. Behavioral Assessment, 4, 1 – 33.

MCTEAR MF (1991) Is there such a thing as a conversational disability?, in Mogford-Bevan K and Sadler J (Eds.) Child Language Disability Volume II: Semantic and Pragmatic Difficulties, Multilingual Matters, 18 – 42.

MEHRABIAN A (1972) Nonverbal Communication. Chicago: Aldine.

MEICHENBAUM D (1975) Enhancing creativity by modifying what subjects say to themselves. American Educational Research Journal, 12, 129 – 45.

MEICHENBAUM D (1977) Cognitive Behavior Modification: An Integrative Approach. New York: Plenum Press.

MICHELSON L, SUGAI D, WOOD R and KAZDIN A (1983) Social Skills Assessment and Training with Children. New York: Plenum.

MITCHELL L (1977) Simple Relaxation: The Physiological Method of Easing Tension. London: Murray.

MOORE S (1967) Correlates of peer acceptance in nursery school children, in Hartup W and Smothergill W (Eds.) The Young Child: Review of Research (Vol. 2). Washington: National Association for the Education of Young Children.

MORENO JL (1953) Who Shall Survive? New York: Beacon House.

MULLINIX SD and GALASSI JP (1981) Deriving the content of social skills training with a verbal response components approach. Behavioural Assessment, 3, 55–66.

NCC GUIDANCE: English in the National Curriculum (No3) (1990) Department of Education and Science: London: HMSO.

NEISSER U (1976) Cognition and Reality. San Francisco: Freeman.

NELSON RO and HAYES SC (1981) Theoretical explanations for reactivity in self monitoring. Behaviour Modification, 5, 3 – 14.

NICHOLS KA (1974) Severe social anxiety. British Journal of Medical Psychology, 47, 301 – 6.

ODOM SL, PETERSON C, McCONNELL S and OSTROSKY M (1990) Eco-behavioral analysis of early education/specialized classroom settings and peer social interaction. Education and Treatment of Children, 13, 316 – 30.

PIAGET J (1932) The Moral Judgment of the Child. New York: Harcourt Brace.

PRIESTLEY P, McGUIRE J, FLEGG D, HEMSLEY V and WELHAM D (1978) Social Skills and Personal Problem Solving. London: Tavistock.

RIMM D and MASTERS J (1979) Behavior Therapy: Techniques and Empirical Findings, 2nd edition. New York: Academic Press.

RINALDI W (1992) Social Use of Language Programme. Windsor: NFER-Nelson.

RINALDI W (1993) Working with Language Impaired Teenages with Moderate Learning Difficulties. ICAN.

RINN RC and MARKLE A (1979) Modification of social skills deficits in children, in Bellack AS and Hersen MH (Eds.) Research and Practice in Social Skills Training. New York: Plenum.

ROFF M, SELLS SB and GOLDEN MM (1972) Social Adjustment and Personality Development in Children. Minneapolis: University of Minnesota Press.

ROSS C and RYAN A (1990) Can I stay in today Miss? Improving the School Playground. Stoke on Trent: Trentham Books.

RUBIN KH and ROSS HS (1982) Introduction: Some reflections on the state of the art: The study of peer relationships and social skills, in Rubin KH and Ross HS (Eds.) Peer Relationships and Social Skills in Childhood. New York: Springer.

RUSTIN L (1984) Intensive Treatment Models for Adolescent Stuttering: A Comparison of Social Skills Training and Speech Fluency Techniques. Unpublished M. Phil. Thesis: Leicester.

RUSTIN L (1987) Assessment and Therapy Programme for Dysfluent Children. London: NFER-Nelson.

RUSTIN L, BOTTERILL G and KELMAN E (1996). Assessment and Therapy for Young Dysfluent Children: Family Interaction. London: Whurr.

RUSTIN L and PURSER H (1984) Intensive treatment models for adolescent stuttering: Social skills versus speech techniques. Proceedings of the XIX Congress of the IALP. London: The College of Speech Therapists.

RUSTIN L, COOK F and SPENCE R (1995) The Management of Stuttering in Adolescence: A Communication Skills Approach. London: Whurr.

SAINATO DM and CARTA JJ (1992) Classroom influences in the development of social competence in young children with disabilities, in Odom SL, McConnell SR and McEvoy MA (Eds.) Social Competence of Young Children with Disabilities: Issues and Strategies for Intervention. Baltimore: Brookes, 93 – 109.

SALTER A (1949) Conditioned Reflex Therapy. New York: Farrar, Straus and Geroux.

SCHEIDT R and SCHAIE K (1978) A taxonomy of situations for an elderly population: General situational criteria. Journal of Gerontology, 33, 848 – 57.

SCHULTZ JH (1969) Übungsheft für das Autogene Training. Konzentrative Selbstentspannung, 14. Auflage. Stuttgart: Thieme.

SHEPHERD G and SPENCE S (1983) Concluding comments, in Spence S and Shepherd G (Eds.) Development in Social Skills Training. London: Academic Press.

SHURE MB and SPIVACK G (1979) Interpersonal cognitive problem solving and primary prevention: Programming for pre-school children and kindergarten children. Journal of Clinical Psychology, 2, 89 – 94.

SPIVACK G AND SHURE MB (1974) Social Adjustment of Young Children: A cognitive approach to solving real-life problems. San Francisco: Jossey-Bass.

STANFORD G and STOATE P (1990) Developing Effective Classroom Groups: A Practical Guide for Teachers. Bristol: Acora Books.

STOBART G (1986) Is integrating the handicapped psychologically defensible?. Bulletin of The British Psychological Society, 39, 1 – 3.

STOKES TF and BAER DM (1977) An implicit technology of generalization. Journal of Applied Behavior Analysis, 10, 349 – 67.

STONEMAN Z, CANTRELL ML and HOOVER-DEMPSEY K (1983) The association between play materials and social behavior in a mainstream preschool: A naturalistic investigation. Journal of Applied Developmental Psychology, 4, 163 – 74.

STRAIN PS and TIMM MA (1974) An experimental analysis of behaviorally disordered preschool children and their classroom peers. Journal of Applied Behavior Analysis, 7, 583 – 90.

STRAVINSKY A (1978) The 'emperor's clothes' revealed or social skills versus research skills. Which are most needed? Behavioural Psychotherapy, 6, 91 – 6.

THORNTON G (1944) The effect of wearing glasses upon judgments of personality traits of persons seen briefly. Journal of Applied Psychology, 28, 203 – 7.

TROWER P (1983) Social skills and applied linguistics: Radical implications in social skills training, in Ellis R and Whittington D (Eds.). New Directions in Social Skills Training. Beckenham: Croom Helm.

TROWER P (1979) Fundamentals of interpersonal behavior: A social–psychological perspective, in Bellack AS and Hersen M (Eds) Research and Practice in Social Social Skills Training. New York: Plenum.

TUCKMAN BW (1965) Developmental sequence in small groups. Psychological Bulletin, 63, 384 – 99.

VYGÖTSKY L (1962) Thought and Language. New York: Wiley.

WALKER HM, McCONNELL S, HOLMES D, TODIS B, WALKER J, GOLDEN N (1983) The Walker Social Skills Curriculum. Texas: Pro-ed.

WEITZMAN E (1992) Learning Language and Loving it: A Guide to Promoting Children's Social and Language Development in Early Childhood Settings. Biscester: Winslow.

WELFORD A (1980) The concept of skill and its application to performance, in Singleton W, Spurgeon P and Stammers R (Eds.) The Analysis of Social Skill. New York: Plenum.

WOLPE J and LAZARUS AA (1966) Behavior Therapy Techniques. New York: Pergamon Press.

WOOD DJ, WOOD HA, GRIFFITHS AJ, HOWARTH SP and HOWARTH CI (1982) The structure of conversations with 6 to 10 year old deaf children. Journal of Child Psychology and Psychiatry, 23, 295 – 308.

YERKES R and DODSON J (1908) The relation of strength of stimulus to rapidity of habit formation. Journal of Compulsive and Neurology Psychology, 18, 459 – 91.

ZIGLER E and PHILLIPS L (1960) Social effectiveness and symptomatic behaviors. Journal of Abnormal and Social Psychology, 61, 231 – 8.

ZIGLER E and PHILLIPS L (1961) Social competence and outcome in psychiatric disorder. Journal of Abnormal and Social Psychology, 63, 264 – 71.

Index